Stress and the Woman's Body

Stress and the Woman's Body

W. David Hager, M.D.

and

Linda Carruth Hager

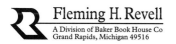Fleming H. Revell
A Division of Baker Book House Co
Grand Rapids, Michigan 49516

Published by Fleming H. Revell
a division of Baker Book House Company
P.O. Box 6287, Grand Rapids, MI 49516-6287

Printed in the United States of America

Library of Congress Cataloging-in-Publication Data

Hager, W. David (William David), 1946–
    Stress and the woman's body / W. David Hager and Linda Carruth Hager.
        p. cm.
    Includes bibliographical references.
    ISBN 0-8007-1717-1 (cloth)
    1. Stress management for women. 2. Women—Health and hygiene. 3. Stress (Physiology) 4. Stress (Psychology) I. Hager, Linda Carruth, 1949– . II. Title.
RA778. H17 1996
613'.04244—dc20   95-36883

Unless otherwise noted, Scripture quotations are from the New American Standard Bible, © the Lockman Foundation 1960, 1962, 1963, 1968, 1971, 1972, 1973, 1975, 1977.

Other versions cited are New International Version (NIV), *The Living Bible* (TLB), and King James Version (KJV).

David: This book is dedicated to all of my patients. Without you, I would not know about stress-related disorders and I would not be able to do what God has called me to—take care of others.

I also dedicate these pages to my wife and children. Without your patience and understanding, I would not have accomplished this task of love.

Linda: I would like to dedicate this book to my spiritual mother and mentor, Margaret Therkelsen. For her example of the fervent, faithful life of prayer, her wise counsel, and her unconditional love I am deeply and eternally grateful.

To David, Philip, Neal, and Jay—thank you for calling me higher up and further into the adventure. You are my most precious jewels.

Contents

Preface

*A*nother book on stress, you say. There are a lot of them out there now. So why should you read this book about women, the stresses they face, and the manifestations of stress in their lives in the form of disease? What is it about this book, which details classic cases of stress-related disorders in women, that will enable you to recognize predisposing factors of disease and avoid them or overcome them? Those are good questions, and we believe that we have the answers for you.

David: I grew up in a busy home and as a child witnessed the response of my mother and sister to stress. I live with a vivacious, active woman who is my wife and the mother of our three sons. Living in what must seem like a men's dormitory is not an easy task for a woman. I have seen the effects of stress on her—in addition to the stresses I have created—and watched as she has learned to cope with them. Linda has experienced problems with premenstrual syndrome, headaches, and fibromyalgia as a result of stress and hormonal changes. Last but not least, I have seen the effects of stress on my patients. Every day in my practice I see women who are devastated by the effects of tension and anxiety. From this fairly extensive experience I will describe many case scenarios so that you may be able to garner information and draw solace and strength to help you on your journey.

Linda: Pressure and strain tend to distort our minds as well as our bodies. Perspective is skewed, and we feel as though we are losing our way along the path of our exterior lives, not to mention our interior life with Christ. Stress is a given in my life as well as yours. This being so, the only relevant question is How can this immovable stumbling block of stress become a building block? As I attempt to deal with my personal battles with narcolepsy, fibromyalgia, premenstrual syndrome, headaches, and the demands of my chosen way of life as a wife and mother I am in the process of coming into a new place where I see answers to my question forming. Whenever the clouds settle and I can see no way out I am learning to own my total lack of ability to push the clouds away. As an act of the will I am turning with increasing regularity to the place of prayer. Through simple conversations with God I tell him about my frustrations and openly admit my anger, my fatigue, my pain. Through the mysterious power of the Holy Spirit, I am finding the consolations of my Savior, Jesus Christ. The ancient mystics teach us that these blessed consolations are found in and through suffering.

"Aren't you overspiritualizing these physical problems?" some may ask. I respond by saying I believe that *all* issues—whether physical, psychological, or emotional—are spiritual at their root. Come along this pathway with me for awhile. Let me walk with you women who, like me, find yourselves under the burden of stress and who deeply, desperately want a way out. I promise you we will never go further than God's grace can take us.

David: I have had to deal with stress in my own life and I have seen its detrimental effects in the lives of men I know. I want men to deal successfully with stress and avoid its consequences, but I agonize for women who deal with these issues. I agonize because I see them every day in my practice of obstetrics and gynecology. It hurts to see women suffer when so much of their pain and agony is avoidable.

For the past fifteen years, I have been a sounding board for my patients. I have listened to stories that were shocking and heart wrenching, emotional and anger provoking. I have had tears stream down my cheeks and fire burn in my gut as these remarkable women have related the events that have molded and shaped their lives.

The stories I have heard are frightening, not so much for the events they convey, but because they are so very frequent that it seems they are epidemic in proportion. Women have described abandonment, abuse, betrayal, illness, death of family members, job pressures, failures, goals achieved, goals missed. Every situation imaginable has been described within the walls of my office. Many of these stresses and the disorders they cause can be prevented by women taking steps to change the circumstances in which they live. When stress is unavoidable they must learn to manage it.

We all have stress in our lives. Even if we escaped to that island paradise we dream about, we would face some stress (hurricanes, sunburn, possibly even boredom). We cannot escape it, but we can learn to recognize it, reduce it, and take steps to avoid its adverse effects. Because Linda and I are Christians, we will direct you toward a personal relationship with Jesus Christ, along with other things you can do to increase the peace and joy in your life.

We want you to be healthy and whole. We don't want the stress you face to destroy your relationships with God, husband, friends, children, or extended family. We will consider the various effects of stress on the female emotions and body. We will look for ways to diminish the causes for disease and decrease the symptoms that trouble women.

Now, you have a choice to make. Most people wait until they suffer the consequences of their behavior before they consider a change in lifestyle. But you can choose to make changes before untoward events occur. Don't wait until you have severe abdominal pain or unremitting headaches before you decide to reduce the stress in your life. Don't wait until you have a heart attack to begin exercising and decreasing your intake of fats. Make changes now.

I ask you to assume that you are my patient, sitting in my consultation office. You have just described your situation at work and home. You have related the symptoms that trouble you and you want to know what can be done about them. I will tell you about the specific causes of the disorder you describe, as well as its symptoms, signs, and treatment. But I will also tell you about other women with similar difficulties (changing their names), to help you realize that others suffer from the same disorder and that there is hope for recovery and relief. So read carefully; you may find yourself on the pages of this book.

It's Monday morning, the start of another work week. Your husband has already left for the office, and you are rushing through the house trying to find Jeremy's tennis shoe. You never have to find both shoes; it is only one that routinely disappears.

"I'm going to be late for work again," you mutter. Finally you find the shoe, but in the meantime Jeremy decides to go fishing in the toilet. After changing his clothes, you bundle him into the car and rush off for the day care center.

As you face the morning rush-hour traffic, you dream about being able to sleep in just one day. Jeremy's unhappy voice pulls you back to reality. "Mommy, my tummy hurts," he whines.

"If you had just taken your time eating your cereal, Jeremy," you bark back at him.

Suddenly your words echo in your mind. "If you had just taken time." The reason Jeremy ate so fast was because you were yelling at him to hurry up while at the same time you were gulping down a donut and orange juice.

After dropping Jeremy off, you head for your job at the insurance claims office. *When are they going to fix that traffic light at Broad Street? I always end up behind someone who pokes along to work.* Your rushing seems to be blocked by the slowness of everybody else. You blow the horn at an elderly man puttering along in his Chrysler New Yorker.

Finally you pull into the company parking lot, jump out of the car, walk double-time to the building, and rush up two flights, pausing to pour a cup of steaming coffee before hurrying into your small, cluttered office. You realize that your head is pounding and your jaw and neck are sore. There is a crampy sensation in your lower left abdomen. You sink into your chair, coffee in hand, and you wonder how much longer you can tolerate this hectic pace.

Your husband asked if you would please cook tonight instead of bringing home fast food for dinner, so you start to prepare a list of the things you will have to pick up at the grocery store. The phone rings and your boss asks you to please run out to one of your large industrial customers who had wind damage to his warehouse last night and prepare an estimate of his losses. You sigh, grab your briefcase, and hurry out the door wishing it were Friday instead of only Monday.

Sound familiar? No, the job or home situation may not be yours, but the chances are that you experience similar or greater stresses in your daily life. You may not experience the tension headache, jaw and neck pain, or abdominal cramps this young woman had, but the chances are that stress reveals itself in some physical form in your body.

Seldom does a day go by that I don't see several patients in my office with various physical disorders that have strong links to stress. It has been estimated that 70 percent of all visits to doctors' offices are for physical or emotional problems that are stress related. Patients frequently are very hesitant to mention the stresses that affect them. They are so focused on the physical symptoms and discomfort they feel that they sometimes even become angry when I suggest, "Perhaps your problems are a result of extraordinary stress in your life." Yet the facts are that stress-related disorders are very prevalent. Tension and migraine headaches, menstrual disorders, irritable bowel syndrome, eating disorders, premenstrual symptoms, fibromyalgia, temporomandibular dysfunction, and substance abuse all have possible associations with stress.

Please don't misinterpret what I am saying. You cannot assume that the symptoms you may be having are totally a result of stress and therefore do not require evaluation by a medical-care provider. Sometimes serious pathology and stress-related ailments have very similar symptoms. Remember, always check with your doctor first. However, if you are told that your symptoms are primarily the result of stress, but you receive no information on how to manage the symptoms and the stress, then find a doctor who will empathize with you and will offer you the help you need.

In this book we use a case scenario format to describe stress-related disorders and what you might do to avoid such clinical problems. The final chapter will describe techniques for stress management, including exercise, dietary change, and spiritual direction. Before we go any further, however, I must emphasize again, not all symptoms that appear to be stress related are. You should always have a careful medical evaluation before assuming that the pain or problem you are having is due to stress. Muscle spasm, headaches, constriction of blood vessels resulting in hypertension can all occur as a result of stress, but serious illness can cause the very same symptoms.

Men certainly have disorders that are stress related. Gastrointestinal disease such as ulcers, cardiovascular disease resulting in heart attack and stroke, and substance abuse resulting in addiction to alcohol and drugs occur much more frequently in males. There are conditions that are more frequently found in women than men, though: migraine headaches, irritable bowel syndrome, anorexia and bulimia, fibromyalgia, temporomandibular disorder, and of course menstrual disorders and premenstrual syndrome.

I believe I can help you understand the fundamental aspects of stress-related disorders because I see these disorders in my practice so frequently. I hear women voice their symptoms and I encourage them to relate to me the stresses in their lives that may be responsible for their disorders. I empathize with them and want to do everything I can to enable them to be symptom free and to lead productive lives.

As a result of these experiences with my patients, I have learned much that I want to pass along to you. Just as I would if you were sitting in my consultation office seeking advice, I want to help you get through this difficult time in your life. You can feel better, be less stressed and more at peace with yourself, with those around you, and with God.

Linda: In the sections called "A Spiritual Perspective," I will be sharing with you the ways I have been learning to access the transforming power of the Holy Spirit as my primary resource for stress management. The calming, healing presence of the Lord transforms seemingly immovable blocks of stress into building blocks that are strengthening my spiritual foundations. At the same time, the Lord is enabling me to deal with tension, pressure, and strain in ways that are redemptive rather than destructive.

You may be nineteen years old with crampy abdominal pain and diarrhea, fifty-two years old with hot flashes, night sweats, and difficulty sleeping, or seventy years old with a recent diagnosis of colon cancer. Whatever your age or circumstances, this book is for you if you are under stress and feel that something has broken, or is about to break, within you.

Acknowledgments

Terry Bourne—Thank you for your tireless efforts in the preparation of this manuscript.

Thank you to the medical professionals who reviewed the information herein for accuracy:

Morris Beebe, M.D.
Timothy Coleman, M.D.
Gregory Erena, M.D.
Laura Humphreys, M.D.
Kenneth Muse, M.D.
Donna Roth, M.D.
Donna Walker, P.T.
Dan Langer, Ed.D.
Pat Soister, B.A.

What Is Stress and How Does It Affect You?

*U*ntil 1950, stress had been defined as "the load that is exerted on a physical structure, such as a bridge or a cross beam." The word was used in physics more than in psychology. In the 1950s, Hans Selye began to define stress in psychological or emotional terms as "the load or tension exerted on individuals, which might alter an individual's ability to respond or react normally."[1]

Before this time, stresses existed, but suddenly it seemed that they were multiplying in a feverish fashion. They came from every direction, and we were not prepared to face them or deal with them adequately—a postwar baby boom, the Korean and Vietnam wars, civil unrest, racial injustice, the information explosion, more competition for jobs, the sexual revolution, changes in moral values, substance abuse, a near-epidemic of sexually transmitted diseases, violence, and on and on and on.

Response to the stresses took the form of social and political reaction but also caused individual emotional, physical, and spiritual reactions. As individuals became more and more stressed, we began to see the physical consequences. Disorders that had never been described before were defined in new medical textbooks.

Along with everything else came another major social change. Women entered the work force. Suddenly, mothers were not just home economists, but they worked outside the home and had to fit their household duties in before and after work. The average woman's work week increased to as much as eighty-five hours, as two-thirds of all married women entered the work force.

What Is Stress?

Juliet Schor indicates that 30 percent of all adults admit high levels of stress. One of every ten Americans suffers from an anxiety-related disorder. Three-fourths of all American women have at least one tension headache a month.[2]

Stress can be defined in several ways. I choose to define it as a state of mental or physical tension or the conditions that induce the tension. Stress can be considered negative if it results in adverse effects in our lives; it can be seen as positive if the end result is beneficial. Indicating that a person is under stress does not necessarily connote an unfavorable situation. I could list many conditions that I would consider stressful, but someone else might consider only one-third of them as being as stressful as I do. Our understanding and conception of pressure, strain, and tension is very subjective. It is safe to say, therefore, that what is negatively stressful for me may be exhilarating or positively stressful for another person.

As we move through our daily lives setting our minds and bodies to the tasks we've been given, a certain amount of stress is inevitable. This will vary with our personality types and the environments in which we find ourselves. Positive stress causes us to move forward and accomplish as a result of the action or force exerted. Negative stress results in reversal and in adverse events and outcomes.

We experience stress from three principal sources: our environments, our bodies, and our thoughts. Environmental stresses include weather, noise, crowding, interpersonal demands, time pressures, performance standards, and threats to our security and self-esteem. Body stresses include illness, accidents, poor nutrition, sleep disturbances, and aging. Mental stress includes our thoughts and imagination.

We perceive stress by sensing the effects on our minds and bodies. Once the stress is perceived, the body demands some form of adjustment to compensate and to diminish stress. If the event previously resulted in pleasant experiences, it will be perceived as less stressful than in events where the result was previously unpleasant. Therefore, it is not just the particular stressor that determines the level of anxiety, but one's prior experience with that stressful event.

Is stress new? No, mental and physical tension have always existed. Based on our current understanding, we may want to say that given situations of earlier eras were not stressful, but when we do so, we forget that much of the reaction and response to stress is based on perception. Before the modernization of medical care, knowing the high death rate from giving birth was stressful and frightening for women. Facing the possibility of infectious disease without the availability of antibiotics or vaccines was stressful. But most stresses for women of past centuries resulted from conditions in and around the home: rearing children, keeping the house clean, preparing meals, raising a garden. The innumerable responsibilities of the home were great, but today women have added the stresses of the away-from-home job world. In essence, women have experienced a doubling of their stress levels. Even if they do not have a second job outside the home, the tensions of our society exert enormous stress.

Another definition that merits our attention is that stress is "a force brought to bear on something, to bring out what is important." In examining this concept of stress, we are brought to an understanding of deeper truths. Our bodies' responses to stress can be red flags alerting us to deeper issues that need to be explored. Self-condemnation is not in order. We must pause to recognize why we find ourselves in these situations and we must then take measures to relieve the negative stress.

Unconditional love should be a gift that we give ourselves. To the extent that we nurture ourselves, we will in turn be able to nurture those around us. Loving our neighbor as ourselves, as God's Word commands, begins with an unconditional acceptance of our own minds, bodies, and emotions, just as we are.

Perhaps a couple is very productive professionally, but their relationship with each other is not what either wants it to be, and they are teetering on the brink of separation. Positively, stress has pushed them to accomplish their professional goals, but negatively, it has damaged their marriage. Unfortunately, stress has brought them to the point of ending their marriage, but it may encourage them to seek counseling and restoration of their relationship. The daily, never-ending pressures of running their home, coordinating their children's schedules and their civic and church duties, plus job responsibilities have put them into an overload or "hot reactor" state. They are on a roller coaster and cannot get off. As a result, they may pay a very high price for their professional success.

On the other hand, the reverse may be true for someone else. A wife may have devoted so much of herself to her husband and children that there is nothing left over for her. She feels empty, angry, and frustrated because of the life choices she has made.

The Effects of Stress

Stresses in life may motivate you to achieve great things, but if stress results in physical illness, you need to change the situation in order to protect your health. Selye and other investigators have shown that stress contributes significantly to the development of disease in animals and humans.[3] Some estimate that 70 to 75 percent of all illness is ultimately stress related.

In order to understand the effects of stress, we must know something of the responses stress causes in the human body. Different personalities recognize and deal with stress in different ways, but potentially we all face the effects of our physical responses to outside stress that destroy us from within.

As early as 1920 physiologist Walter Cannon described the fight or flight response to stress in humans. All societies have had a perception of stress, but never has so much stress affected so many people. Who can say that the stress of climbing the corporate ladder is greater than the stress generated by the fear of wild animals lurking just outside the cabin? But we are stressed more relentlessly today. The "animal" we face is not a living beast. It is pressure and tension. No matter what the stress, the result is a bodily response to fight or flee.

Fight or flight does not mean that some are brave and fight and others are frightened and flee. It is a reaction that occurs as a stressed person chooses to fight, to destroy the offending stress, or to escape the cause of stress. By lowering the stress level, a woman can lower the levels of hormones secreted into her body's systems. Those hormones, responses to stress, evoke specific stress-related effects.

Though we no longer fear wild animals or an invading tribe, we are concerned about that job promotion or about safety in the inner city. As we have developed as a society, the number of stressful events in our lives has increased—as a result, the possibility of adverse effects on our body systems has also increased.

In their book, *Is It Worth Dying For?* Robert Eliot and Dennis Breo describe the scientific methods used to measure the way the body responds to stress—the way it functions, its chemical responses, and its observable responses. The body secretes into the bloodstream chemicals that have effects on all our body systems. Among the changes are increased heart rate, elevated blood pressure, and increased contractility—pumping action—of the heart. The blood supply to muscles and sense organs is increased. These responses occur to prepare the body for fight or flight.

Neil Hibler has described the emotional, behavioral, and physical signs of stress for us.

Emotional Signs

Apathy—the blahs, feelings of sadness, lack of pleasure in recreation

Anxiety—restlessness, agitation, insecurity, sense of worthlessness

Irritability—hypersensitivity, defensiveness, arrogance, argumentativeness, rebellion, anger

Mental fatigue—preoccupation, difficulty concentrating, trouble thinking flexibly

Overcompensation or denial—grandiosity (exaggerating the importance of your activities to yourself and others), workaholism, denial of problems, ignoring of symptoms, feeling suspicion

Behavioral Signs

Avoidance—keeping to yourself, avoiding work, neglecting or not accepting responsibility

Doing things to the extreme—alcoholism, gambling, drugs, sexual promiscuity, spending

Administrative problems—tardiness, poor appearance, poor hygiene, accident-prone

Legal problems—indebtedness, traffic tickets, uncontrolled rage

Physical Signs

Phobias about illness or denial of illness when it exists

Frequent sickness

Physical exhaustion

Reliance on self-medication, overuse of drugstore remedies

Ailments—headaches, insomnia, changes in appetite, significant weight gain or loss, indigestion, nausea, diarrhea, constipation, menstrual disorders, sexual dysfunction, muscle and joint pains and aches[4]

Natural Defense Mechanisms

Before I describe individual disease states that are frequently stress related, we must understand the body's natural defense mechanisms.

The body is created to be able to respond to physical demands and stresses. These events result in one of two responses: alarm or vigilance. Alarm has to do with the body's immediate reaction to stressors. Vigilance concerns preparation to face the long haul of a stressful event. The adrenal glands, small glands that rest atop each kidney, produce chemicals—hormones—that are secreted into the bloodstream to stimulate responses in body systems. The alarm reaction is brought about by adrenaline produced by the adrenal glands; the vigilance reaction is caused by cortisol (natural steroids), produced in the same area. Eliot and Breo describe these two reactions.[5]

Alarm is an emergency reaction to prepare us for fight or flight. It is an acute reaction to stress that enables us to speed to another's rescue, pull a child from a burning building, prepare for a surprise quiz, fight off a physical attack, resuscitate a fallen victim on the street.

In this normal bodily response, adrenaline pours into the bloodstream from the adrenals; the heart increases in its rate of contraction and in its pumping efficiency; blood pressure rises, and blood is shunted from areas of low energy need, such as the skin, stomach, and kidneys, to areas of high energy need, such as the heart, lungs, brain, and skeletal muscles.

The changes of the alarm reaction result in other changes that we associate with panic or anxiety. The pupils dilate, the face flushes as blood vessels in the skin dilate, the rate of breathing increases. In addition, the liver releases fats into the bloodstream to provide a quick source of energy. Glucose and other sugars are released into the bloodstream, along with more insulin to promote movement of the sugars into cells. All of these changes occur several times a day as we respond to stressful events. These events may include rushing to get ready, preparing mentally for the events of the day, driving in rush-hour traffic, getting a speeding ticket, or being involved in an accident. Other events may include disagreements with the boss or another employee, being frustrated in checkout lines or fast-food restaurants, the children forgetting their homework assignments until the last minute, financial crises, sudden illness, and debilitation or death of a family member.

Vigilance is the withdrawal system of the body that prepares us for long-term survival in the face of scarce nutritional resources. In essence, this is a survival response to loss of control by the individual.

The vigilance response is brought about by cortisol, produced by the adrenal glands. As a result of this survival mode, the blood pressure increases slowly; tissues in the body retain sodium; high-energy fats and agents to promote the clotting of blood are released; production of sex hormones is suppressed so as not to compete with energy for vigilance; there is an increase in acid produced by the stomach; the immune system is altered so that resistance to disease is suppressed; there is difficulty sleeping.

Vigilance may occur on an infrequent or on a daily basis. Infrequent occurrences would include working variable shifts with altered sleep patterns, heavy seasonal work, stressful overtime sessions at work, or a death in the family.

Daily occurrences might include a problem child, an abusive husband, the pressure of a regular job outside the home plus daily preparation of meals and housekeeping, chronic financial worries, or spiritual division within the home.

Now that you understand the way in which the body was designed to respond to stress by fight or flight, consider what happens when neither fight nor flight is an option. It is not acceptable to slug your boss or run out the back door at home and never stop running. You have to stay and see these stresses through to some resolution, even though your body has prepared to fight or flee. The chemicals are in the bloodstream and must have an effect. Eliot and Breo term this age-old phenomenon *uncoupling*. The body is prepared to act and react; however, no battle occurs, and the stress effects are rendered against the body itself.[6]

Another term for this type of reaction is the *freeze response*. The body prepares for fight or flight, but when those responses aren't socially acceptable, a freeze may occur. In this situation, the victim of undue stress may actually deny that extreme tension exists. If we deny it, then we reason that we won't have to face the consequences stress exerts on the body and the mind. As a matter of fact, the effects may be even more devastating to us when we are in a freeze response. The self-destruction from uncoupling or freezing results in many of the stress-related diseases you will read about in this book.

In the following chapters, I hope you will be able to identify with one or more of the case scenarios described. The names have been changed to protect my patients' identities, but the cases are real-life examples of how destructive stress can be to the body, mind, and soul. You will be reminded again and again of the powerful effects of stress. I want you to know about these disorders so that you can recognize them if you are suffering from their symptoms. My intent is not to frighten you, but to make you more aware, so you can make appropriate changes in your life to reduce the disabling effects of stress.

There is a strong spiritual emphasis in each chapter on managing stress—not an emphasis on one's own self-healing capacity, but an emphasis on the restorative power of Jesus Christ in one's life. I remind you that Jesus existed before time began; therefore, he is not bound by time. Yet he became, in human form, a part of our timed existence. He knows what it is to feel the effects of time. He assumed on the cross all of the sinful effects of our time so we would not have to bear them anymore. We carry the effects of our past and present stresses into the future, sometimes resulting in illness. Jesus is saying, in effect, "Leave the past with me. I paid the price so that you can be free of those negative results in the future." As Jahaziel the prophet told Jehoshaphat in 2 Chronicles 20:15, "the battle is not yours but God's."

A Spiritual Perspective

I once read a story about a professional pilot who worked for the National Weather Service. It was her job to fly head-on into violent thunderstorms. With her plane shaking, she looked for an opening in the dark, boiling clouds. This crevice in the cloud structure enabled her to fly into the eye of the storm. While there, she collected valuable data and tracked the progress of the storm for the Weather Service. She said that the eye was so peaceful one could scarcely believe fierce and dangerous weather surrounded it.

We pilot our personal ships through many rough places, hoping to arrive at a peaceful center. Sometimes there are maladjustments in our spiritual lives, leading to increased and unnecessary pressure that batters our vessels until we wonder if we'll survive to reach that peaceful center.

The Old Testament records that when the one true God chose to reveal himself to the Hebrews, the core of that revelation centered around his demand that they serve and worship only him. They were to look to him alone for their identity. His jealousy was not an expression of a dysfunctional emotion but a demand for singleness of worship. That demand has not been revised over time. Why would God be so rigid on this point? Whatever gets the best hours of our days owns the deepest places in our hearts. What is deepest in our hearts will eventually have full dominion over our bodies and minds. Our bodies will begin to manifest the agendas of our minds. God created us in his own image, and part of the meaning of that is that we find in him alone our true and full identity. It is to our detriment that we attach our hearts to anything or anyone but him.

For example, I can honestly say that I love our three sons more than my own life. But as dear and precious as these guys are, they make very poor objects of worship. If I allow their plans and my desires for their success to be what I live for, I have turned my children into idols. If I teach them that they are the center of the universe, I do them and myself no good.

Such pseudolove is an expression of fear and insecurity— if I don't give them everything they want, will they still like me? If they fail or aren't happy, is my identity as a good and successful parent at stake? How much do I depend on the approval of my children and on their success for validation? But if I am finding my identity in Christ, I will be a better parent and I will not suffer the stress of a driven, fearful spirit.

Here is another example. As the natural aging process manifests itself in my body and on my face, what is my response? The answer to the question will tell me a lot about how much I have depended on youth and looks for validation. The fear I feel will shape the way I spend my time and handle the financial resources God has placed in my stewardship. Do I create stress in my life, perhaps even overextending myself financially, in a vain attempt to purchase approval? Does my physical being reflect rebellion and fear? Or does a deepening inner peace of trust in God soften the wrinkles and brighten my face?

John 14:27 teaches us that Jesus gives us a kind of peace that is nothing like what the world has to offer. Are you interested in getting in on his offer? How interested are you? What price are you willing to pay for the peace Jesus wants to give you? No one can answer that question for you. Nothing but obedience can purchase the peace of Jesus for you. I cannot tell you what he will ask you to do to find this peace, but I know he has a plan that is custom-tailored for you and your circumstances. Don't let anyone but Jesus tell you how to live your life.

Scriptures for Meditation

Isaiah 8:13–18

As you read these verses, begin to do some thinking about *who* and *what* you regard as "holy." To regard someone or something as holy means that you consider that person or thing worthy of all of your attention, time, and reverence. To regard as holy means that you believe that person or thing has the power to change you for the better, in ways that will be most conducive to your happiness.

Some of the things to which we may attribute life-changing power are wealth, prestige, and recognition (by everyone with whom we come in contact) of our success, beauty, intelligence, sensuality, or social elitism—the list is endless and very subjective. Quite often this is a hidden agenda born of early life experiences and buried deep in our subconscious minds. The power these agendas have over us is rooted in the very fact of their hiddenness. It takes fierce personal honesty in prayer to begin to uproot these troublesome agendas.

To whom does the Word of God attribute life-changing power? Does this knowledge alter your perspective? If so, how? why? In light of this knowledge where should you place your trust?

Isaiah 55

This Scripture always reminds me of my tendency to try to draw water from dry wells. I shop, I eat, I perform, I run errands—all in an attempt to find fulfillment. Others may jog, study, or throw themselves into work. While these activities are not inherently sinful, the point is this: They will never be able to permanently quench the thirst of our spiritual selves.

Can you identify some "dry wells" in your life? Could some of the stress in your life actually be disguised forms of spiritual hunger? If so, are your current efforts to deal with this stress producing peace of mind and a calm spirit?

A Suggested Prayer

Dear Jesus, I am so tired. My weariness goes all the way to the bone. Even when I sleep, I wake up exhausted. I am worried about so many things. Sometimes it is hard for me to believe that you care, but I choose to believe that you understand even my doubts and that you love me in the midst of them.

My schedule is so packed with important things, and I can't imagine giving up even one of them. Help! Will you really show me where to put my left foot and my right? Will you really get that intimately involved in my life? Lord, I want to believe; help my unbelief. Give me a heart that hungers and thirsts to know you, even more than I hunger and thirst for rest and peace. When I want to know and understand you more than anything else in my world, I will have come to the beginning of the end of stress that threatens to undo me. Reveal yourself to me, Lord, and I will follow. Amen.

2

The Stress of Abuse

*C*urrent estimates show that one of three women and one of seven men in the United States were sexually abused before they were eighteen years of age. In a recent office survey, we found that 41.8 percent of all the women who walk through the door as patients have been abused in some fashion. Of those, 59.5 percent admit to sexual abuse, 60.8 percent to verbal abuse, and 41.8 percent to physical abuse. Among all those women, only 29 percent had received counseling.

Because abuse and its effects are too common, and taking steps to resolve the psychological scars of abuse occurs too infrequently, I've chosen to begin my consideration of stress with this topic.

The Psychological Impact

Abuse has a devastating psychological impact on the victim. Dean G. Kilpatrick indicates that the psychological symptoms reported by victims of crime (which include abuse) are consistent with the diagnosis of post-traumatic stress disorder (PTSD) or major depression. PTSD is defined as an acute psychological reaction to an inordinately stressful event that has been experienced or witnessed. Three groups of symptoms are required to make the diagnosis: re-experiencing, avoidance, and arousal.

Re-experiencing the event includes having distressing nightmares, flashbacks, and intrusive thoughts about the traumatic event. Avoidance involves the trauma victim's deliberate attempts to avoid any reminders of the traumatic event. These reminders may include situations and people related to the event, or simply talking or thinking about the event in general.

Arousal in trauma victims may manifest itself as hypervigilance, irritability, difficulty concentrating, shortness of breath, palpitations, or difficulty falling asleep or staying asleep.[1]

Rates of PTSD for victims of crime vary from 24–25 percent for individuals sampled from community-based studies, to 48.4–70 percent for more indigent populations. In the first two weeks post-crime, Rothbaum found that 94 percent of rape victims met the full criteria of symptoms for PTSD. At three months post-crime, 47 percent still met full criteria. Kilpatrick, Veronen, and Resnick reported that 61 percent of rape victims who sought treatment for rape-related PTSD an average of eight years after the crimes also met criteria for a major depressive disorder.[2]

But there is hope for abuse survivors, as you will see from Grace's story.

"It took a long time before I could allow myself to recall the abusive events of my childhood, but when I did, they came rushing back like a runaway locomotive," Grace told me. "I could see myself asleep in the room that I shared with my older sister: white sheets, a down comforter, and my favorite ragged pillow. I was sound asleep.

"But then something disturbed my slumber. There is one sound, and then another. The sound of footsteps, tiptoeing yet heavy, moving from one room to the next. Footsteps in the kitchen, in the hallway, in my doorway, a doorway that has no door, just a curtain.

"I try to go back to sleep, praying that it's only a bad dream. But sleep is gone. No dream, but a terrible reality shatters my night. It begins again, as it has so many times before. I am haunted by its memory.

"The sound of his breathing. The sound of a zipper opening. The rustling. The breathing. The sound of flesh rubbing against flesh, almost slapping at times, getting faster and faster. The breathing becomes labored, and there is this awful lip-smacking noise. I don't have to see it to know what it is. I've heard it, seen it, awakened to it, been exposed to it, what seems like hundreds of times."

Grace has been awakened from her childhood slumber, from her innocent dreamland, and thrust into a vile, contaminated adult world. She has been robbed of her right to an innocent childhood, robbed of her right to feel good inside, to have good thoughts about herself.

"I know, without looking, that my father stands there, penis in hand, staring at me. Digesting my little body with his eyes. Whether I pretend he is there or not, he persists, beating out a rhythm on his body that I don't understand. Sometimes he stands aloof; sometimes he touches me. I don't know why, I don't know what it all means. I whimper. I cry.

"I stir, turn over as if I were waking up, in hopes that he will go away. Sometimes it works, sometimes it doesn't. I don't really know what to do. If I scream, will he hurt me, or will he run away? It must be my fault, something I do that makes him come at me this way. I feel powerless, worthless, dirty, hopeless.

"I want to be invisible. I want to escape. I must escape. I let my mind take me to another place, a place that is a safe haven from these harsh realities of life. I separate myself from this situation, and from these people.

"Quickly I learn that if I lie perfectly still and don't resist the probing and prodding, his breathing will eventually slow down, and he'll go away for a while. I learn to adapt, to acquiesce, to be someone I am not, but there is so much that I don't understand. Am I supposed to understand this?"

During her early thirties Grace became depressed. Eating and sleeping were almost impossible. When she did sleep, she experienced frightening nightmares.

Sometimes the nightmares took on physical reality. One night, she awakened from a nightmare to find herself standing at the bedroom window, beating it as hard as she could with her fist. In her dream, her father was outside the window masturbating, and she was determined to break the glass to get to him and kill him.

In addition to the nightmares, there were frightening flashbacks of the abuse. Grace feared that she was losing her senses and would never return to the world of sanity. Her attention span was short. Concentration on work or activities at home was extremely difficult. A constant gnawing pain in her stomach and loss of appetite led to significant weight loss. Anxiety seemed to permeate her existence.

The effects extended to others. Friendships became strained, and many were broken. Although she tried to date, it was all pretense. There was no depth to any relationship. Grace couldn't connect, couldn't trust anyone, couldn't reveal her inner, shattered self.

"Most of the time, I couldn't stand to be touched by anyone," she said. "A certain way that a man would touch me or look at me would immediately trigger a flashback of something my father had done. I didn't feel safe enough with anyone to share these flashbacks, these feelings, these achings of my heart. Anytime a person tried to befriend me or reach out to me, I could only see my father blocking the door of escape from my room. It was as if he were there, panting, exposing, heaving, and preventing me from leaving."

Grace found that her standby coping mechanisms of repression, suppression, denial, and dissociation were no longer working. Feelings of being worthless, hopeless, powerless, dirty, guilty, angry, sad, distrustful, and lonely replaced any positive feelings she had ever had. She felt that she was in the bottom of a deep, dark pit and could not climb out. Suicide seemed to be the only escape from this dark hole. At least she would be transported somewhere, she reasoned. God would understand her pain.

A suicide attempt requiring hospitalization initiated a turnaround. "I woke up to a life I didn't want to live but found myself surrounded and comforted by friends. I became aware of my need for God and found him reaching out to me to lift me out of that bottomless pit. Only divine arms could lift me out of such a place.

"In therapy, I began to see who I was—a victim; not an instigator, not a seducer, not dirty or bad. I learned that I could trust other people and that many others were survivors just like me. Slowly I returned to the world of others and away from the dark, lonely world of myself. I wasn't worthless but had value. I wasn't hopeless but had a future. I wasn't powerless but had a voice. I could breathe again. He could not hurt me anymore.

"Then the anger came. I hated every rotten, evil molecule of his being. I had to get it out. I drew pictures, hit pillows, yelled and screamed and cried. Oh, how I cried for that part of me that was taken away. My little girl who was hurt and couldn't tell anyone about it. My childhood that was shortened by an adult who used me to satisfy his continual pursuit of power and control. I cried out and called him every name I could think of. How could he do this to me, his own daughter?

"Every night I would cry myself to sleep. But slowly those tears began to dry. Slowly a smile came to my face. My appetite returned. I found that I could enjoy my friends. I went back to school and found that I could learn again. People were interested in me again. Socialization had to be in groups at first. I still couldn't trust a man alone.

"Resolution of the physical consequences of my abuse came as slowly as the emotional. Menstrual irregularity continued for some time. The cramping and bloating of irritable bowel syndrome still troubles me. Migraine headaches can be disabling at times, but now that I know these disorders are stress related, I can begin to seek resolution of the stress so that I will feel better physically."

Grace is on the road to emotional, physical, and spiritual well-being. She continues in counseling, has a strong group of dedicated friends, holds an excellent job, and is working on the issue of confronting her father.

But what about the other one-third of the female population who have experienced similar life-changing abuses? We live in a day where revelation of abuses of all types is more acceptable than in the past. Yet many women either have no conscious awareness of their abuse or still do not feel comfortable seeking help to resolve the traumatic consequences. If you are such a person, I encourage you to take the first difficult step along the road to recovery by trusting someone who can help you with your hidden secret. Don't let the darkness victimize you any longer.

Behavior and Personality Changes

If you've suffered from abuse, the trauma has had a powerful impact on the way you think about and react to your world.

In her book *Trauma and Recovery,* Judith Herman says that repeated trauma in adult life erodes the structure of the personality already formed, but repeated trauma in childhood actually forms and deforms the developing personality.

She goes on to say that the pathological environment of childhood abuse forces the development of extraordinary capacities, both creative and destructive. It fosters the development of abnormal states of consciousness in which the ordinary relations of body and mind, reality and imagination, knowledge and memory no longer hold. In order to survive emotionally, the victim must do whatever is necessary. She feels that she must take control of her own survival. This may take the form of repression and amnesia, dissociation, depersonalization, or multiple personalities.[3]

In the abused individual, the normal regulation of bodily functions is often disrupted. In this out-of-control state, the victim may manifest eating disorders, gastrointestinal complaints, sleep disorders, habitual lying, stealing, gambling, excessive spending, workaholism, self-mutilation, and suicide attempts. These responses are survival techniques for the desperate.

As mentioned earlier, the responses of the abused fall into a diagnostic category of PTSD. This disorder results in the alteration of various aspects of one's behavior and personality.

Alterations of self-perception include shame, guilt, and self-blame. Alterations of consciousness, which are attempts to separate emotionally from the trauma, include amnesia of the events and various forms of dissociation and depersonalization. Multiple personalities can result from this dissociation.

There may be alterations of effect, including unhappiness, self-injury, imagining suicide, anger, and sexual inhibition. Self-injury may progress from minor damage to mutilation. Suicidal thinking and gestures may lead to attempts at self-destruction. Sexual inhibitions may result in extreme frigidity and avoidance of any heterosexual relationships. Homosexual relationships may be perceived as the only safe sexual encounters.

Anger builds in the abuse survivor until it begins to destroy from within. The emotion is directed toward everyone, including the victim herself. Anger is a normal response to abuse, but frequently the nature of the relationship with the abuser prevents appropriate expression of the emotion toward him or her, and the feelings are inappropriately refocused on others. The anger needs to be redirected in an appropriate manner toward the perpetrator so the victim can deal with it effectively, attempt to work toward anger resolution, and try to forgive.

Alterations in relations with others can result in an encompassing fear of intimacy with anyone. The victim has no desire to reveal any aspect of the real self, for fear of being betrayed. Since she was confronted and abused by a false self, she may learn to only reveal her false self. Isolation and withdrawal frequently occur.

There may also be alterations in the perception of the perpetrator. The abused person may assign unrealistic power to the abuser and may actually experience a sense of a supernatural relationship and a mixture of fear and admiration. There is always an underlying fear of being violated and hurt—hurt physically, yes, but also hurt to the depth of the soul.

The Recovery Process

Recovery from abuse is a long, arduous process. First, recognition and identification of the abuse must occur. Then, in-depth counseling must begin. All the emotions must be dealt with, and the victim must come to see herself as just that, a victim—not an instigator or a seducer, but an innocent victim of the expression of another's illness. Then, and only then, can she begin to emerge as a survivor.

Perhaps the best way to describe this process is in the words of Grace herself. "My recovery is about who I was then, who I am now, and who I am becoming. I now understand that there is no one medicine or therapy style or exercise that one can use to recover. There is a process at work, and it is different for everyone. It feels as if it is going to take forever, and in fact, it is lengthy. There are no shortcuts. It takes as long as it takes. Therapy is about trial and error, facing issues, hard work, pain, and persistence. It is about faith when you feel that you possess none and about hope when all hope seems to have vanished. It is about love when the love has been sucked from your heart.

"I gained strength from facing issues that I once avoided. As I conquered these emotional monsters [shame, guilt, self-blame, and fear] one at a time, I found assurance that I could win another battle. Working through this process has helped quiet my inner turmoil. It has taken some of the edge off the rage I harbored for so long. It has been like defusing a bomb that, once, could explode at any time but now cannot kill me. The abuse no longer has the power and control it once had.

"Working through the process has enabled me to explore places inside myself that were once too frightening to enter. I faced the pain, rage, and grief, and in some instances, relived them; but this time I had God's help and a different perspective. I found positive, cathartic results. My greatest grief is for the little girl who could have been, but who had her childhood taken away."

In their book, *The Courage to Heal,* Ellen Bass and Laura Davis describe the grieving that must be done in abuse recovery. They indicate that repressed grief poisons a person, limiting her capacity for joy, spontaneity, and life. If you were an abused child or adolescent, you may have had to repress your feelings when it was normal and appropriate to be expressing them. If you are like many, you may have even fantasized that your childhood was good. Now you must relive the experience with an adult perspective, grieve for it, recognize that you are safe now, and allow healing to occur.

Bass and Davis detail the grieving that must be done. You must grieve for the child—yourself—who was hurt, for your loss of feelings, for the abandonment you suffered, for your past and present state, for the damage and the time it takes to heal, for relationships ruined and pleasures missed.[4]

Dealing with the grief and doing appropriate grief work will, as in Grace's experience, lead to anger. When the anger is appropriately dealt with, you can begin to put the pieces of your life back together. The strength gained from a well-grounded commitment to God is irreplaceable. You cannot recover alone. The indwelling Spirit of God will come alongside you and enable you in your journey to recovery. His desire is for you to be whole—your little girl of the past, the woman of the present, and the person you are becoming.

Perhaps you have read the information in this chapter, heard Grace's story, and recognize that you need help in this area of your life. What do you do? Let me offer some suggestions.

You have overcome the first hurdle in recognizing that there is a problem. The first thing I recommend that you do is read. Even before you seek counseling or perhaps before you confide in a trusted friend, read. Reading empowers you because you gain knowledge about abuse beyond your particular situation. With this new understanding, you will be better able to ask appropriate questions of those you choose as counselors or confidants.

Start with a book by Eliana Gill, *Outgrowing the Pain.* You will find questions and comments that will help you determine where you are in the process. Then go to *The Right to Innocence* by Beverly Engel and then *The Courage to Heal: A Guide for Women Survivors of Childhood Sexual Abuse* by Ellen Bass and Laura Davis. Beginning to read about abuse is the first step to recovery. Before recovery actually begins and mental health is stabilized, take the necessary steps to ensure your safety from the perpetrator of the abuse and from yourself, recognizing that the depression often suffered by a victim has the potential to encourage self-harm.

Seek help. You may want to begin with a friend, your minister or priest, or with a counselor. Where can you go for help? Some suggestions include a comprehensive care center, a church support group, a spouse-abuse center, a rape crisis center. Most states and larger communities have councils on child abuse that can offer assistance and get you plugged into the program that is right for you. Some cities have a child advocacy center to allow for interviews of the abused outside of a police-station situation.

Now the process begins. Remember that there will be ups and downs. It is going to be hard work, but it will be the best work you ever do. Therapy will begin with further recognition of the problem. There will be time to mourn and grieve your losses. Remember that facing the pain is the only way to get to the other side. None of us likes pain. We want to turn and run from it, but you must walk through the fire to get to healing. There will be times of depression and falling back, but slowly you will become less passive in your therapy and more active. It is a long process—trust it.

As you begin to see healing, I would encourage you to write your feelings down. You may want to share your story, as Grace has done, and eventually you will want to reach out and help others. Your focus will turn from the internal to the external. You will feel more comfortable in group therapy. Remember that in all of this pain and processing, God understands your grief.

God invites you to come to him. It may take time for you to trust your relationship with him, but he is faithful and true and is trustworthy. He wants you to be restored. He is a God of love. He can even help you forgive what seems unforgivable.

As you deal with the issues of abuse and resolve them, you will find that your stress-related disorders begin to decrease in their severity. Headaches, muscle and joint pain, bowel symptoms, abnormal menstrual periods will slowly resolve, and you will be whole again.

Anger may flare up within you whenever you are reminded of the past. Remember, God can accept your anger. He understands the cause of all emotions. You can take it to him and allow it to be defused as you express your hostility. He can be your safe harbor. You can learn that God is the safest one with whom you may express your intimate thoughts. You can survive.

> But Jesus said, "Let the children alone, and do not hinder them from coming to Me; for the Kingdom of heaven belongs to such as these."
>
> Matthew 19:14

> But whoever causes one of these little ones who believe in Me to stumble, it is better for him that a heavy millstone be hung around his neck, and that he be drowned in the depth of the sea.
>
> Matthew 18:6

A Spiritual Perspective

"All truth is God's truth, wherever you find it." Have you ever heard that saying before? Some theologians debate it, but I see more and more evidence of its validity. Nowhere do I see it more profoundly articulated than in teaching aimed toward abuse recovery. Let me explain.

The most dangerous thing a Christian can do is to compartmentalize her life into categories of Christian truth and secular truth. The Word of God is either relevant to every life issue we face, or it is not relevant at all. What is required is a discerning heart tuned to the voice of the Holy Spirit. How is such a heart acquired? Through time spent daily in conversant prayer and in the reading of the Word. No truth given to us by the Holy Spirit will be contradicted in his Word. With this in mind, take the information you receive from any and all sources and apply the Scriptures to it. God's Word is the ultimate truth. He understands your pain and wants you to be whole again.

Scripture for Meditation

1 Corinthians 2:12–16

It takes the Spirit of God to understand the mind of God. As Christians we have access to God's Spirit. In the original Greek versions of the New Testament the Spirit of God is referred to as the *parakletos* of God, that is, the one who stands alongside of God and acts as his helper. The prefix *para* also implies protection against. From this simple lesson in word origins we can better understand the office of the Holy Spirit as a part of the triune (three persons in one) nature of Almighty God. He is our helper and protector. Is your understanding of what God wants to provide for you personally beginning to expand?

As you read the suggested verses, reflect on your particular situation. Envision the *parakletos* of God standing right beside you. You may want to write down a list of ways in which you would like the Holy Spirit to help you. Begin actively watching with your spiritual eyes and listening with your spiritual ears for his answers, his teaching that is just for you and your situation. Check your intuitions against the Word of God, remembering that what he speaks to your heart will never be in conflict with what he reveals in his written Word.

A Suggested Prayer

Blessed Holy Spirit, I ask you today to give me the mind of Christ concerning all that I have been taught by my counselors and all that I have read from sources outside of your Word. Help me to open my deep inner person to your work, Holy Spirit, so that I may more readily hear and understand your voice and receive your truth, dear Lord, wherever you may choose to show it to me.

3

Premenstrual Syndrome

Seldom a day goes by in my practice of gynecology that I don't see a woman with symptoms consistent with premenstrual syndrome (PMS).

Perhaps one reason that some people doubt that PMS exists is because of the diversity of symptoms. Although the symptoms vary, the common denominator is the timing of the symptoms in the menstrual cycle. The following three patients' case histories will emphasize the variation in changes that occur.

Carolyn was referred to my office for evaluation by her psychiatrist. In a referral note, he indicated that he had been seeing Carolyn for over a year and had seen very little improvement in her condition. The psychiatrist wanted to know whether there might be a hormonal connection to her behavior.

Based on the referring physician's notes, I expected to see a barely functional woman. Instead, a very nattily dressed, intelligent, perceptive one sat in my office. She immediately stated, "Perhaps it would have been better if I had come in when I am in the midst of my symptoms, rather than when I am feeling good."

"What do you mean?" I questioned.

"Well, I'm thirty-six now. When I was about thirty-three, I began to notice some changes in my behavior. I had been a salesperson for a large marketing firm here. When my husband and I decided to have a family, I quit work. I had two daughters within the space of three years and did not return to work. We were very happy to be parents, and our marriage was great, but I never realized what great pressure is involved in being a wife and in being a mother of toddlers," she said.

"Sometimes I am just fine, but at other times I become less and less able to function," Carolyn explained. "I get so depressed that I feel overwhelmed by everything. Just getting the girls up, dressing and feeding them, and preparing breakfast for my husband is more than I can handle some days."

I still had not commented, so Carolyn continued to relate her history. "John, my husband, was the first to notice it," she said as she began to cry.

"Notice what?" I asked.

"At times I am, as he calls it, my good old self; there are other times when he doesn't recognize me because of my behavior. He is very loving and tries to help me in every way he can, but it hasn't seemed to make a difference. Finally, things got so bad I had to seek professional help.

"Dr. Hager, I'm a Christian, and I have a solid relationship with God; but at times, I feel that something has actually come in and possessed me," she blurted out with a sob. "Things will be going along fine, and then I start to get depressed. I feel worthless. My self-esteem, which has always been great, becomes nonexistent. I have insatiable cravings for chocolate and sweets. I feel bloated and puffy. Headaches become more frequent. I become irritable; even the smallest thing, like a messy diaper, can send me off. John never knew who to expect at home, until he figured out that I am this way only for two weeks before my period; after my period starts, I am fine. I can't believe it took a man to figure that out, but it just got by me.

"My psychiatrist tried to treat the symptoms with a sedative, but it doesn't consistently make me better," Carolyn complained. "I want to feel better all month, not just for half of it. He referred me to you to see if this really can be hormonal. What do you think?"

"You have given me a lot of information, Carolyn," I replied. "Although I can't be certain, your symptoms may fall into the diagnostic category of premenstrual syndrome.

"We don't know the exact cause of PMS, nor do we know exactly how to treat it; but one thing is certain, the symptoms occur repeatedly prior to the menstrual period and end rather abruptly with the onset of the period or right after it is over."

"I feel as if I have to have help right away, Doctor," Carolyn pleaded. "I considered taking an overdose of sleeping pills during my last episode of depression, although I know that I really couldn't kill myself."

"Did you actually have sleeping pills at home?"

"No, and as I said, I really don't think I could have taken them."

I gave her a symptom calendar to mark with the timing and nature of her symptoms on a monthly basis. She said, "I can fill this out right now. I know exactly what is going to happen and when each month."

"That may be true but recording your symptoms as they occur will give us the most accurate picture."

I tried to reassure Carolyn that I would try to help her: "Although we don't know the specific cause and therefore specific treatment, there are some things that we can do to help you feel better and regain control of your life."

Irritability was a major problem in Carolyn's collection of symptoms. Even though she complained of headaches, swelling, and a chocolate craving, irritability and depression had the greatest effect on her day-to-day life and were impacting her family and friends.

Rhonda, a twenty-five-year-old woman whom I saw in the office for a routine gynecologic visit, had a very different history. In the course of my conversation with her, I discovered that she had been released from four jobs in the past eighteen months. When I inquired about the reasons for her failure to hold a job, Rhonda replied, "I don't know what happens to me, but at certain times, I become angry with everyone around me, and I cannot control my temper. It seems that no one can do anything right."

During these periods of extreme anxiety and bursts of anger, Rhonda would lash out at anyone who did not please her. Fellow employees and customers became the victims of her outbursts. Rhonda's employers would talk with her about controlling her emotions, but after a brief respite, the episodes would recur, and she would be fired.

In reviewing these events with her, it became obvious that Rhonda's tirades always occurred the week before her period. She would become extremely anxious, develop bloating and swelling, and eat constantly, especially chocolate. Though she would vow not to allow the angry outbursts to happen, she seemed to have no control over them. She explained, "I'm always sorry for the way I act, for the fact that I hurt people so much with my anger. I get focused on myself, and I can't consider anyone else. I'm not satisfied with who I am, and I want to bring everyone else down too."

The third woman, Andrea, is a thirty-two-year-old mother of three children. We had talked in the office previously about PMS when she complained of irritability, mood swings, and bloating before her periods. On this visit, however, Andrea was distraught. She burst into tears as she described an event that had occurred recently, ten days before her period.

She was preparing the evening meal while her three-year-old and six-year-old played in the den. The children were shrieking and laughing. Andrea asked them to stop making so much noise. When her order was not promptly obeyed, she stormed into the den, smacked her six-year-old, and grabbed the three-year-old and threw him against a chair. The child screamed in fear and began to whimper as he lay stunned on the floor. Andrea ran to her room, fell on the bed, and sobbed.

Andrea's husband came home from work to find the children crying and the den a wreck. He questioned Andrea about what had happened, and she lashed out at him about daring to come home and attack her when she had been closeted at home with two children all day. She left the house and didn't return until late that night.

When she returned, she expressed dismay about her behavior. She apologized to the children and to her husband, but they could not understand when she told them that it wasn't really her. They were frightened and confused by her actions. Her husband insisted that she see a doctor immediately.

"You're not yourself," he said. "Please find out if something is wrong."

Although these three stories are different, they have a common thread. Sometime between the middle of the menstrual cycle and the onset of a period, these women felt that they lost control of their lives, and their behavior was radically changed.

Normally, these women function as well-adjusted members of society. Suddenly, at midcycle or shortly thereafter, symptoms begin to occur; there is a drastic change in mood, and their ability to exert control over their behavior is altered. Not just some, but many aspects of their behavior are affected. They struggle just to get from one day to the next without hurting themselves or those around them.

Yes, there are various degrees of severity of PMS-related symptoms. Some women experience what is termed *premenstrual tension*. They go through a certain degree of anxiety and an uncomfortable mood change, but it's not enough to cause them to seek medical care. Others experience more severe symptoms, but with medical advice and their own resilience, they are able to get through each month without disintegrating. The cases that you have just read are among the worst, with symptoms including consideration of suicide, repetitive uncontrollable outbursts of anger, and difficulty getting along with others.

A Medical Understanding of PMS

The syndrome was originally described as a constellation of findings that focused on the premenstrual phase of the cycle and caused varying degrees of debilitation in women. These findings include both physical and behavioral changes. Occurrence of the symptoms after ovulation and before the end of menstrual flow is the key to diagnosis. Accurately diagnosing this syndrome is difficult. Many patients may be treated for PMS when they should have a different diagnosis (and vice versa).

The most comprehensive definition of PMS is that proposed by Reid and Yen, which describes PMS as "the cyclic recurrence in the luteal phase [latter part] of the menstrual cycle of a combination of distressing physical, psychological, and/or behavioral changes of sufficient severity to result in deterioration of interpersonal relationships and/or interference with normal activities."[1]

Some writers want to include a condition called premenstrual magnification syndrome (PMM) as a form of PMS. In premenstrual magnification syndrome, symptoms occur throughout the menstrual cycle but consistently increase in severity during the premenstrual phase. Because the findings do not meet Reid and Yen's definition of occurrence of symptoms in the latter phase of the cycle, PMM cannot be considered a type of PMS.

Catamenial disorders are a type of PMS. These disorders are categorized as single, specific problems that occur in the premenstrual phase of the cycle, such as migraine headaches, seizures, or rashes.

The American Psychiatric Association defines psychiatric disorders in its *Diagnostic and Statistical Manual* (DSM). In the latest revision, DSM-IV, the term *premenstrual dysphoric disorder* (PMDD) is used instead of PMS. Premenstrual dysphoric disorder is classified under mood disorders—depression not otherwise specified. The unfortunate thing about such a classification is that it indicates that women with PMS have a mental disorder. Although some women with PMS may have an underlying psychological disorder, most have physical and/or behavioral changes without associated psychiatric illness. Because you may see a physician or psychiatrist who uses this DSM-IV classification system, it is important to understand that perspective. Although I agree with 1, 2, 4, and 5 below, the symptoms listed under 3 have not all been derived from empirical data.

The latest DSM-IV criteria for the diagnosis of PMDD state:

1. In most menstrual cycles during the past year, symptoms occurred during the last week of the luteal phase and remitted within a few days after the onset of the follicular phase. In menstruating women, these phases correspond to the week before, and a few days after, the onset of menses. (In nonmenstruating women who have undergone hysterectomy, the timing of luteal and follicular phases may require measurement of circulating reproductive hormones.)
2. The disturbance seriously interferes with work or usual social activities and relationships with others.

3. At least five of the following symptoms have been present for most of the time during each symptomatic late luteal phase with at least one of these symptoms being either a, b, c, or d.
   a. Marked affective lability (e.g., feeling suddenly sad or tearful)
   b. Persistent marked anger or irritability
   c. Marked anxiety, tension, and feelings of being "keyed up" or "on edge"
   d. Markedly depressed mood, feelings of hopelessness, or self-deprecating thoughts
   e. Decreased interest in usual activities (e.g., work, friends, hobbies)
   f. Lethargy, easy fatigability, or marked lack of energy
   g. Subjective sense of difficulty in concentrating
   h. Marked change in appetite (e.g., overeating, specific food cravings)
   i. Hypersomnia or insomnia
   j. Other physical symptoms (e.g., breast tenderness or swelling, headaches, joint or muscle pain, bloating, weight gain)
   k. Avoidance of social activities (e.g., staying at home)
   l. Decreased productivity and efficiency at work and at home
   m. Increased sensitivity to rejection
   n. Subjective sense of being overwhelmed
   o. Subjective sense of feeling "out of control"
   p. Increased interpersonal conflicts
4. The disturbance is not merely an exacerbation of the symptoms of another disorder, such as major depressive disorder, panic disorder, dysthymic disorder, or a personality disorder (although it may be superimposed on any of these disorders).
5. Criteria 1, 2, 3, and 4 are confirmed by prospective daily self-ratings during at least two symptomatic cycles. (The diagnosis may be made provisionally prior to this confirmation.)[2]

There are many different opinions about the existence of PMS. If you are one of its victims, you can attest to the fact that there is definitely a constellation of symptoms that occur in a cyclical fashion and that they may be severe.

Data are variable concerning the influence of stress on PMS, although most researchers feel that there is a correlation. Beck and Gannon indicate that stress per se does not cause PMS, but it does magnify or increase the severity of symptoms.[3] Heilbrun, on the other hand, states that stress and personality (especially self-preoccupation) are sensitizing factors for PMS.[4]

Carol Tavris, in *The Mismeasure of Women,* incensed that women are labeled with PMS, writes, "Why are we so willing to believe our hormones make us weepy, bitchy and unreliable? The latest word is that very few women have a monthly problem . . . and that real equality means never having to say you're premenstrual."[5]

Although I understand the political implications of such a statement, as a practicing gynecologist, I see so many women with cyclical complaints consistent with PMS that I am convinced it is a describable syndrome. It is estimated that 4–7 percent of reproductive-age women have symptoms consistent with PMS. However, these are only the worst cases. In my practice, at least 20 percent of premenopausal women admit to some PMS-related symptoms. Many women have symptoms that are secondary to normal hormonal cycling and are not purely PMS related. These include fluid retention, minimal weight gain, food cravings, breast tenderness, and painful periods.

The symptoms attributed to PMS include both physical and behavioral changes. Among them are anger, anxiety, bloating and weight gain, breast swelling and tenderness, clumsiness, constipation, depression and sadness or hopelessness, decreased alertness or concentration, decreased self-esteem, decreased interest in usual activities, decreased libido, swelling of the hands or feet, fatigue or lethargy, food craving or overeating, gastrointestinal complaints, headache or migraine, impulsivity, irritability, agitation or listlessness, mood swings, muscle and joint pain, and sleep disturbances and tension. Once again, the key to attaching these symptoms to the diagnosis is that they occur between midcycle and onset of the menstrual period, and they are repetitive. Some women have one or two symptoms, some women have many. One of two basic patterns usually makes up the PMS constellation; either depression, or anxiety and tension seem to dominate. In taking a history, it is important to determine which pattern is dominant.

Where depression exists, I have found that most patients experience an underlying low-level anger. Some express this with a comment such as, "I've always been angry," while others may say something like, "Ever since I married Bob, I've struggled with anger." In such cases, I advise my patients to seek counseling to unearth the hidden causes of their emotions.

History is the key to making a diagnosis of PMS. Keeping a symptom calendar to determine the time in the cycle when the physical and emotional changes occur is recommended. Begin to keep a calendar on which you record any symptoms you have and take it with you when you see your physician. Keeping a record for three months should be sufficient.

As you read the list of symptoms, perhaps only three or four caught your attention as complaints that you routinely have. That's not unusual. Most women have a few of the symptoms, but those symptoms do recur regularly with each cycle. It is unusual to have varying complaints each month or for the symptoms to occur at varying times. Most women note that their physical and behavioral changes occur on approximately the same days of each cycle. The severity of the symptoms may not be as important as the timing.

What Causes PMS?

I wish I could tell you that there is one specific cause for PMS and that we are working on a cure for that cause, but I cannot. Many theories have been advanced, but still no definite origin has been determined.

Women secrete two principle hormones from their ovaries, estrogen and progesterone. Even if only one normal ovary is present, adequate amounts of the two hormones are produced. Estrogen is the dominant hormone of the early part of the menstrual cycle. Estrogen stimulates the inner lining of the uterus (the endometrium) to grow and thicken. Ovulation, the passage of the egg from the ovary, usually occurs at midcycle or approximately day fourteen. A shorter or longer cycle may be normal for certain women. After ovulation, progesterone becomes the dominant hormone, causing further thickening of the endometrium, along with an increase in blood vessels to support the potential implantation and growth of a fertilized egg. When fertilization does not occur, the cycle proceeds to a menstrual period.

We do know that PMS probably is not related to the change in hormone levels that occurs in a woman's body before menstruation. Well-designed scientific studies have not been able to determine specific excesses or deficiencies in estrogen or progesterone. However, we also know that PMS occurs only when the ovaries are functioning to make both estrogen and progesterone, that the disorder is detected only in women between puberty and menopause, and that postmenopausal women do not have PMS. Women who take hormonal replacement in menopause may have some PMS symptoms.

When considering a diagnosis of PMS, it is important to rule out certain specific disorders that may have some symptoms similar to the syndrome. These include psychiatric problems such as unipolar and bipolar disorders, anxiety neurosis, and personality disorders; problems of the pituitary, thyroid, or adrenal glands; anorexia/bulimia; and chronic fatigue state.

Treatment

Because we do not know the cause of PMS, it is difficult to determine a specific treatment of the syndrome. There is no specific, scientifically proven treatment for PMS that everyone accepts. Many nonprescription and prescription medications have been tried. Suppression of estrogen and progesterone by medications, which suppress the brain's production of stimulating hormones, just as occurs with menopause, seem to diminish PMS symptoms. The problem is that evoking early menopause in order to treat PMS may have more negative than positive effects. Use of antidepressants also appears to benefit PMS sufferers. At present, we can only say that some interventions may have benefits for PMS.

Exercise is very important for the PMS patient. Regular, moderate exercise acts to relieve stress, which PMS often causes, and also promotes release of beta endorphins (natural pain relievers) into the bloodstream. Four studies have associated PMS with altered beta endorphin levels. Unfortunately, treatment with these substances has resulted in variable effects.

No specific dietary changes have been shown to effectively help or cure women suffering from PMS. Restriction of refined sugar, salt, caffeine, and chocolate has been evaluated, but with no consistently beneficial results.

No specific elements or minerals are consistently deficient in PMS sufferers. Calcium and magnesium have both been used in treatment regimens, and two recent studies have reported possible benefits from supplemental magnesium given from ovulation (midcycle) until the onset of the period. As with many other studies, it is difficult to show any greater benefit from these forms of treatment than from placebo treatment.

Stress reduction has not consistently been proven beneficial in relieving PMS symptoms, but meditation, contemplation, and reduction of job-related anxieties often help relieve symptoms. It is important, however, that the PMS sufferer not become so preoccupied with her symptoms that she neglect her overall health. Eating appropriately, exercising, stimulating the mind, staying occupied with others, and receiving spiritual direction are important. Many women say that when PMS strikes, they cannot think of anything except how miserable they are. This is where an understanding physician or counselor, as well as the devoted love of a friend or spouse, is crucial. Do not hesitate to describe your symptoms to someone close to you; if you do not get an appropriate response, get him or her some literature on the subject.

The use of diuretics (water pills) to treat premenstrual bloating has been reported in several studies. The symptoms of bloating, swelling, and weight gain from fluid retention may be improved with a diuretic like spironolactone, but this should only be used for short periods of time each month. This prescription drug must be taken only under a doctor's order.

Recent work has focused on sleep manipulation to benefit PMS sufferers. Advancing or delaying sleep may have an impact on mood disorders. Melatonin, a hormone that is increased in the presence of light, affects darkening of the skin and has some feedback effects on the regulation of the menstrual cycle. Using light therapy to change melatonin levels is being studied to determine its effects on mood, but statistically significant benefits have not been shown. An article in the *American Journal of Psychiatry* reported on a study in which fourteen PMS sufferers had their symptoms recorded for two months. These women were then given light therapy for two hours a day, during the week prior to menses. (The theory is that light restores the body's normal circadian rhythms by stimulating melatonin release in the brain.) Among those who received treatment, the study reported a 38 to 66 percent decrease in the symptoms of depression.[6]

Some frequently used forms of treatment have never been scientifically proven to be beneficial. Vitamin supplementation with B6 or B-complex may have some effect on hormone levels but does not affect mood. Vitamin A is not effective in treating PMS. The use of natural progesterone in either a vaginal suppository or in an oral micronized form has been touted by Dalton and others, but once again, predictable benefits have not been proven. Treatment has been from midcycle until the period begins. Birth control pills have no reliably beneficial effect on the syndrome. Twenty-five percent of pill users improved, 50 percent had no change, and 25 percent worsened. Placebo medications have had a significant beneficial effect in altering symptoms. This focuses attention back to the psychologic overlay associated with PMS and makes the evaluation of other therapies difficult.

Successful Treatment

Some specific medications have shown promise in relieving symptoms. Danocrine is an androgen (male hormone) that can relieve PMS symptoms; it successfully blocks ovulation and normal menstrual cycles. Danocrine will also relieve the symptoms of painful breasts. Because it is a male hormone, side effects may include hair growth, increased appetite, weight gain, and liver problems. Patients must consider these before initiating treatment.

Psychoactive medications, or antidepressants, have been used with great success. These include: fluoxetine, Buspirone, Alprazolam, sertraline hydrochloride, and fluoxetine hydrochloride.

A form of therapy that has been investigated in well-designed studies is gonadotropin-releasing hormone agonists (GnRH). Feedback to the brain results in a menopauselike effect. All physical and psychological symptoms resolve within a month of initiating injections, and relief persists as long as treatment continues. These preparations are expensive, as is danocrine. Because they cause cessation of estrogen and progesterone production, menopausal effects such as hot flashes, night sweats, and vaginal dryness may occur. One of the side effects that can occur is bone breakdown (osteoporosis). Also, cardiovascular problems may occur. Therapy is usually limited to six months, to avoid bone damage. The use of additive estrogen and progesterone while on GnRH may help prevent or lessen this problem.

Management of PMS

Treatments with Proven Benefit	Treatments without Proven Benefit	Treatments with Possible Proven Benefit
Regular exercise	Diet—avoiding caffeine, chocolate, refined sugar	Magnesium
Antidepressant therapy		Placebo
GnRh agonist therapy	Vitamin supplements	
Danocrine	Diuretics	
Stress reduction	Progesterone therapy	
Psychoactive medications	Birth-control pills	

Regardless of the medication(s) prescribed for you, it is key to have an understanding medical provider and support from friends and family. You must be willing to exercise regularly in order to have any chance of getting better. Some form of treatment may help your best friend but not you. Keep trying until you find the treatment that benefits you.

Carolyn, the young woman who considered suicide, continued in counseling and had a dramatic improvement in her symptoms with the initiation of an exercise program and antidepressant therapy.

Rhonda was treated with exercise, spironolactone, and danocrine. She showed no improvement in her symptoms and was referred to a psychologist for counseling to address her inability to keep a job.

Andrea, who had abused her children, was placed in counseling by the police department. She responded to the initiation of an aerobic exercise program plus an antidepressant. She later began counseling with a marriage and family specialist. At the time of her last appointment with me, she was amazed at the remarkable change in her moods and behavior; her marriage was on the mend.

PMS is an enigma. We do not know its cause. We have some forms of treatment, but few appear definitely better than a placebo. We continue to try different forms of management for different patients to try to relieve their sometimes incapacitating symptoms. The key is to continue searching for the lifestyle changes and medication that diminish your symptoms. Quiet time in meditation will help you to dissipate the stress that results from your PMS symptoms.

A Spiritual Perspective

One of my most precious memories stems from a day in my life when I was in the full throes of PMS, and I raged against one of my small sons for some minor offense. Immediately afterward, the Holy Spirit moved my heart with deep remorse. I called my little boy to my side. He came reluctantly. How it grieved me to see my own precious baby moving in fear of me. I took his small hands in mine and said, "Sweet pea, I should not have yelled at you like that. You have not done anything wrong. I don't feel good in my body, and I am taking it out on you. Will you please forgive me?"

His little face reflected genuine concern for me, and he said, "Mama, I want to think about it before I forgive you."

I asked him to sit down beside me, and I prayed a simple prayer that went something like this, "Lord, please forgive me for hurting my son, and help him to forgive me when he is ready. Thank you for the love that we share with each other."

He got up and went off to play. In about an hour he came and found me. "Mama," he said, "I'm ready to forgive you now." I scooped him up in my arms, and we held on tightly to each other as I acknowledged my wrong and received his forgiveness.

A few days later, I was still feeling bad, and he came to me of his own volition. He asked me to sit down, and he put his little hands on either side of my forehead. "Do you want me to pray for you?" he asked. "I think you need it." How can anger and ugliness stand in the face of such innocence and sweetness? Gladly, I received his prayers on my behalf. That child is now six feet tall, and we walk in deep love toward each other. Prayer stood in the gap, and repentance removed the sting of my wounding behavior.

Some of what rears its ugly head in our cyclic depression is garbage that has been pressed down deep into our psyches. Whatever the physical impetus for the onset of PMS, the syndrome serves to peel back the layers of our psychic wounds, and the worst in us comes forward.

In our culture it is not popular to attach any positive significance to the emotion of guilt. Many teachers, particularly those involved with New Age thought, teach the eradication of all guilt, as if by removing it we nullify the negative consequences of choices made out of our dark side. Zechariah 10:2 teaches us that when comfort comes out of deceit it is comfort given in vain, and the result is a people who "wander like sheep oppressed for lack of a shepherd" (NIV).

When we verbally, emotionally, or physically abuse our families or other people for any reason, the guilt we feel cannot and should not be ignored. Being able to do wrong and feel right is an indication of serious mental illness. To do wrong, for any reason, and feel wrong about it is an indication that our true Shepherd is active in our lives. Answer his call to repentance.

Get all of the medical help that is available for PMS. Follow the advice on total health care recommended in this book, and do not fail to address the spiritual ramifications of this problem. To do so is to miss the opportunity for some priceless lessons in your life in Christ. In our late twenties and early thirties we set the stage for midlife crisis or for midlife renewal. If we are to move toward maturity, we must begin as early as possible to be very intentional about our journey with Jesus. We prove our intentions when we allow every circumstance of our lives to drive us toward him.

Scriptures for Meditation

Romans 5:1–11

Once I became fully aware of my own capacity to do wrong and to inflict deep pain on people I claimed to love, I realized I would have to walk in repentance *daily,* if not *hourly.* Since that terrible revelation, I have never been able to forget what a debtor to grace and mercy I am. Yet through Jesus I am able to be set into right relationship first of all with my heavenly Father—my sin doesn't have to be a permanent barrier between me and the love of God. The blood of Christ was spilled for *me*—not when I became good enough to merit this sacrifice but *while I was yet a sinner!* (see verse 8).

Because of the reconciliation that the blood of Jesus makes possible between me and the heavenly Father I am also able to be reconciled to my human family when pain has created a wall between us.

On your worst days have you hurt the people you genuinely love? I have. It makes me sick when I yell and scream and lose control. I see the pain in the faces of my loved ones and I want so much to say, *Wait! This isn't really* me. *My body is being taken over by hormones and it's all out of control. Help! Somebody, please help me hold it all together and stop this raging.*

But you know what? If I dig way down into my emotions I have to admit that there is a dark part of me that also *enjoys* letting my temper have control. The loud voice, the cutting words, they feel like a cathartic for all my tension. I am actually thinking, *Why should I suffer alone? I feel bad so let's spread it around!* Then as the words hit like bullets and the screams cut like hot blades on tender flesh, the awful reality of the consequences of my unstrung fury hits my gut and I am sick. I am sick because I see with everyone else my sinful, willful, hateful dark self. I can't take it back; I can't cover it up. I can act like I don't care and walk off the battlefield, leaving the wounded to fend for themselves or I can literally fall to my knees and say to my precious ones: "This is wrong. I am out of control and it's nobody's fault but my own. Please forgive me. this is not the way I want to be. Please ask the Lord to help me. I love you all too much to go on hurting you like this."

1 Corinthians 10:13

When you feel overwhelmed with tension and frustration and your last nerve just got stepped on, what way out will you find?

2 Corinthians 1:21–22

When the Spirit of God comes into our hearts he pours himself over us as a shield, a covering. This is what it means "to be anointed." It is the anointing that breaks the yoke. Think of the yokes that are placed across the shoulders and around the necks of cattle or draft horses. These yokes are meant to keep the animals in a state of subjection to their master. Likewise, we become yoked to bad attitudes, bad habits, and anger. We become the slave and the bad stuff becomes the master and begins to link us to our dark side. It takes the anointing of the Holy Spirit to break these yokes.

Have you ever asked for the anointing of the Holy Spirit? Is the Spirit of God living in your heart? What evidence do you have of this?

Galatians 5:1

What part does your will play in your spiritual battles? Do you choose the attitudes you have or are you the victim of the attitudes that have you?

What does this verse in Galatians say to you about experiencing victory over circumstances?

Ephesians 6:11

If you were invited to go on a hike through rough terrain would you wear your high-heeled shoes and an ankle-length silk dress? You wouldn't because you know you would never make it through the hike. You might even be injured because you were not properly dressed. Likewise, we may face serious spiritual injury, and in these days even physical harm, if we move out into the world without the proper spiritual attire.

According to this passage from Ephesians what is the proper spiritual attire? What is the function of this special clothing? What do you risk without it?

Suggested Spiritual Exercise

Take the children to Mother's Morning Out, or to the baby-sitter's, or to a friend. Find a quiet place where you can be alone and uninterrupted. Honor Jesus by speaking honestly and openly with him. Trust his unconditional love. He will never shame or reject you. Look up each of the verses listed above, then ask the Holy Spirit what he wants to teach you from the Word. Ask him how to apply the words of Scripture to your deep inner wounds. Ask the Holy Spirit to show you how to access his supernatural grace and strength on your worst PMS days. Ask Jesus to enable you to walk in deep love and repentance when you fail. Receive the fullness of his love and forgiveness for you.

4

Menstrual Disorders

Sixteen-year-old Kim was brought to my office by her mother because the teen had stopped having periods. Kim had had the onset of normal periods at twelve years of age. After she experienced regular monthly periods for four years, suddenly her cycles became abnormal.

As Kim and her mother sat in my consultation office, it was obvious that the young girl was troubled. Her mother answered every question for her and repeatedly emphasized how busy Kim was, trying to make good grades so that she could be accepted by a prestigious girls' school. Later I found out from Kim that she had been told, "You must make As and high Bs in order to be accepted into college." Daily her mother reminded her of this and put a great deal of pressure on her.

Shortly after completing her college selection visits, Kim had the onset of irregular periods with some spotting between periods. Then her periods stopped altogether. Kim's pregnancy test was negative, and all other lab work was normal. I prescribed a progesterone medication for her, and three days after completing the treatment, she started a normal period.

Kim's cessation of periods occurred in conjunction with her mother's pronouncement about the necessity of superb grades. Though Kim denied being stressed, the level of her anxiety was obvious by the way she behaved in the office.

"Would you mind going to the waiting room while I talk with Kim alone?" I asked Kim's mother. When her mother left the room, the young woman fidgeted in her seat and could not look me in the eye. I knew that some barriers would have to be broken before we could communicate effectively.

"All I want to do is help you during this difficult time in your life," I said.

Kim replied, "I just wish everybody would leave me alone. I'll be just fine."

"Why do you think people won't leave you alone, Kim?"

Kim hesitated and then said with difficulty, "I don't know. It's like my mother wants to be me. She wants me to do things and be things that she couldn't. She wants me to dress the way she tells me, go out with boys she likes, wear the perfume that she picks out. She wants me to make all As but won't tell me what her grades were in school. She wants me to be a cheerleader and enter talent and beauty pageants. It just seems that I can never do enough or be enough."

By this time, the girl was crying. I handed her a box of tissues and said, "Kim, you only have to be who you want to be. God tells us that we can be complete in him, not in your mother or your father or anyone else, but in him. I'll talk with your mother because she may not realize how much stress she is placing on you. I know that she loves you and wants the very best for you. She needs to find her own security, instead of finding it in you."

Disorders of the menstrual cycle are the third leading cause of visits to gynecologists' offices, exceeded only by vaginal infections and family planning. These disorders don't just include delayed onset of periods in the very young and irregular bleeding in the woman about to go through menopause; they include problems across the reproductive age range.

The Normal Menstrual Cycle

In order to understand abnormal menstrual function, you must first know about the normal menstrual cycle. The endometrium is the inner lining of the uterus that builds up during the normal cycle and is then shed in the menstrual period. The normal cycle lasts approximately twenty-eight days, with ovulation occurring at approximately day fourteen or fifteen. There are two principal hormones involved in a woman's menstrual cycle: estrogen and progesterone.

In the normal cycle, estrogen and progesterone affect many organs, but the focus of their effects is on the endometrium. The normal cycle is controlled by these two hormones, produced in varying amounts over the twenty-eight days. Estrogen causes the lining of the uterus to grow and thicken, beginning on about day five of the cycle, with day one being the first day of menstrual bleeding. Ovulation occurs on approximately day fourteen. After ovulation, progesterone begins to be produced in increasing amounts, and along with estrogen, causes the lining of the uterus to swell and thicken even more in preparation for the possible implantation of a fertilized egg.

If intercourse has occurred within the narrow twenty-four- to thirty-six-hour window of possible conception at midcycle, sperm may meet the egg in the fallopian tube, and fertilization may occur. The fertilized egg will begin to divide and, in about six days, will implant in the prepared lining of the uterus. Continued production of estrogen and progesterone signal the brain that further ovulation is unnecessary, and no further periods occur.

If the egg is not fertilized, it will pass into the uterus and eventually be shed with the menstrual blood. The estrogen and progesterone levels decrease, resulting in no further thickening of the uterine lining, and it is shed on about day twenty-eight as the normal menstrual cycle begins.

Two principal hormones produced in the brain affect ovarian function. *Follicle stimulating hormone* (FSH) promotes development of pockets—follicles—in the ovaries, in which eggs develop. *Luteinizing hormone* (LH) stimulates the ovary to release an egg. Alteration of these hormones cannot only affect ovulation but normal cycling.

Numerous studies have shown a relationship between stress and abnormal menstrual function. Due to hormonal differences, women respond to stress differently than men. Not only do pulse and blood pressure increase, but clotting factors are altered, and hormones such as adrenaline are released in increased amounts. These hormones can interact with hormones such as LH and FSH (produced in the brain, in the hypothalamus) and prolactin (produced in the pituitary gland), to interfere with normal ovulation. Therefore, stress can definitely play a role in infertility. Stress resulting in dietary changes and changes in normal daily functions can alter normal menstrual function.

As we discuss various cases of altered menstrual function, remember these basic principles.

In Kim's situation, stress had caused hormonal changes that resulted in absence of normal ovulation and no periods. How these changes occur is not known precisely. We do know that a definite link exists between emotions and the menstrual cycle. The central control area for both of these responses is the hypothalamus. When the hypothalamus does not release LH and FSH, ovulation does not occur, and either periods are missed or irregular bleeding occurs.

As part of my responsibilities in obstetrics and gynecology at the University of Kentucky, I provide gynecologic care for the female athletes. One of the most frequent reasons for me to be consulted by the trainers and team physicians is to treat menstrual disorders. Although women in any sport can develop menstrual dysfunction from the stress they are under to succeed, I see these problems more frequently in long-distance runners and gymnasts.

The onset of normal periods is intimately related to a girl's percent body fat and the ratio of her height and weight. Each female has a thermostat if you will, that is located in the brain. This "thermostat" triggers the beginning of menstruation at a particular height/weight ratio for that individual.

Early rigorous training in childhood may not allow an athlete to achieve the amount of body fat that results in enough weight to allow her to begin having periods.

Candace was nineteen years old when I first saw her as a patient. She had started running competitively when she was eight years old and had never started her menstrual cycle. She was referred by the team's orthopedist because she had a severe stress fracture in her lower leg. She was not ovulating, and her estrogen level was abnormally low. Estrogen is involved in the process of keeping calcium in bones and thus keeping them strong. As a result of her low estrogen level, Candace had developed osteoporosis, which led to her susceptibility to stress fractures. Since she did not want to stop running competitively, I started her on birth control pills to provide the estrogen that she needed to strengthen her bones, and after allowing the stress fracture to heal for nine months, she was able to run again without pain.

Most athletes start vigorous training after they start normal periods and then find that their percent body fat is reduced by the rigor of exercise. Their periods stop.

Renee is a gymnast who was striving to earn a place on the Olympic team. Renee was working out extensively, which is stressful enough, but she also had a great deal of self-induced emotional stress out of her desire to succeed. She came to see me because her menstrual cycles were very irregular. She might go four months without a period and then have spotting for three weeks. Obviously this was an inconvenience to her in competition because she never knew when her period might begin. Cycling Renee with oral contraceptives allowed her to control her periods and also helped strengthen her bones.

The discussion of these cases is not intended to discourage you from exercising physically or mentally. Moderate exercise is beneficial in keeping fit, controlling weight, and reducing stress. When done in excess, however, it may cause bodily changes that are detrimental to your health.

Kim, the sixteen-year-old whom we discussed at the beginning of the chapter, was not an athlete but experienced the same result of stress, the cessation of periods. No matter what the cause of stress (emotional, nutritional, or as a result of strenuous physical exercise), the outcome may be inability to begin having periods or interruption of normal periods.

Kim did not want to take a birth control pill to regulate her menstrual cycle. She did take progesterone for ten days each month, and monthly periods began again. The key to her therapy, however, was counseling for Kim and her parents so that the stress was diminished. When Kim's mother understood what she was doing to her daughter, the pressure to excel academically decreased, and Kim resumed menstrual periods without progesterone.

Although the leading cause of no periods in young women is pregnancy and a major cause of irregular or abnormal periods is stress, pathologic causes of abnormal periods must always be considered before a diagnosis is made.

Brenda, a thirty-eight-year-old mother of three, came to see me with complaints of severe pelvic pressure and excessive bleeding with her periods, to the extent that she was anemic. Brenda was very fearful that she might have cancer. Examination revealed an extremely enlarged uterus with irregular masses in it. These masses are commonly called fibroids. Because of the size of the fibroids, the excessive bleeding, and the fact that she had previously had tubal sterilization, Brenda was scheduled for a hysterectomy. I treated her with a medication that acts to temporarily decrease the size of the masses so that surgery is less difficult. She then underwent a hysterectomy and has recovered completely.

Several other disorders can cause abnormal bleeding. How do you know when to report abnormal bleeding to your doctor? When periods are heavy enough to cause anemia (low red blood cell count), last more than seven days, occur more frequently than every twenty-one days, or when there is bleeding between normal periods, you should see your doctor, who will evaluate you and determine if testing is indicated. Also, remember the importance of having regular Pap smears.

Menopause

Menstrual disorders in women of reproductive age frequently result from stress. Menopause, on the other hand, is a normal event that doesn't result from stress, but frequently causes significant stress in women of that age range. It is appropriate then to address menopause in any book on stress in women.

The word *menopause* conjures up many different perceptions for women and for men. Most of the thoughts that you have about menstrual periods in general came from your mother or the woman involved in raising you. Your image of what it is like to go through menopause comes from your recollection of what it was like living with Mom during that time. Fortunately many of the adverse symptoms that women of previous generations had to suffer can now be altered with hormonal treatment.

Menopause is that time in a woman's life when her ovaries stop producing enough estrogen and progesterone so that menstrual periods cease. The average age of menopause in the United States is 51.3 years and has increased slowly over time. The time when you become menopausal may vary considerably from that age, however. Occasionally, a woman may have premature menopause (ovarian failure) as early as twenty-five to thirty years of age. On the other end of the spectrum, I have had patients who were still having normal menses at fifty-five or fifty-six years of age. There is a tendency for menopause to occur at approximately the same age in families, but even that can vary. The time just before menopause begins is called the perimenopausal period. During this time, many of the symptoms of menopause may begin, yet periods continue to occur, even though they may not be regular.

When women are younger, their periods usually occur in a fairly dependable cycle, flow is moderate to heavy (unless you are on birth-control pills), and the period begins and ends abruptly. As women age, it is not unusual to become somewhat less regular. Some spotting before the onset of normal flow is not unusual. Cramping may become more intense, and occasionally a cycle will be missed. You may also feel the discomfort of ovulation more frequently as you get older.

Stress can result in abnormal cycles and thus abnormal or dysfunctional bleeding. Dysfunctional bleeding is related to hormonal alterations, whereas abnormal bleeding refers to bleeding caused by abnormal conditions such as fibroid tumors in the uterine wall, or polyps in the uterine lining (see the following table).

Causes of Abnormal Bleeding from the Uterus

Bleeding Due to Hormonal Imbalance	Bleeding Due to Pathologic Conditions
Excessive emotional stress	Fibroids. Noncancerous, smooth muscle growths that form on the outside of the uterus, within its muscle, or on the inner lining
Nutritional factors	
Excessive exercise	
Hormonal problems from thyroid disease	Adenomyosis. Benign growth and thickening of the uterus
	Polyps. Usually benign growths off the inner uterine lining
	Uterine or cervical cancer
	Problems resulting from birth-control pills or hormonal replacement
	Endometrial hyperplasia. Abnormal growth and thickening of the uterine lining

The principal symptoms of menopause result from lack of estrogen's effects on the nervous system and on the body's tissues. Hot flashes, night sweats, dryness in the vagina, difficulty sleeping, and irritability are the most frequent complaints heard. Sometimes these symptoms will

occur at a much earlier age than fifty, and you will need to
be evaluated by your doctor to see if you are menopausal.
A blood test that measures follicle stimulating hormone
can tell if your ovaries are no longer functioning at normal
capacity; it is better known as an FSH test.

Barbara was forty-seven years old when I saw her as a
patient for the first time. She had put off going to a doctor
for several months because her mother told her that she was
going through the change, and if she would just be patient,
the symptoms would resolve. "After all, they did for me, and
I never had to take those dreaded hormones." Barbara's
complaints of hot flashes, night sweats, severe mood changes,
and irritability continued for six months. Finally, she had had
enough, and she made an appointment.

It was obvious from Barbara's symptoms what her diagnosis was. An examination revealed a slight decrease in breast
size from a year ago and also vaginal dryness and irritation.
I explained to her what she already knew, that she was
menopausal. Most of her symptoms could be reduced or
resolved with hormonal replacement, in the form of estrogen
and progesterone, I told her. Then I explained the potential
risks as well as the benefits, and she had to decide whether
or not to initiate replacement therapy.

Estrogen can be administered in the form of a pill, in
the form of a patch attached to the skin, or in the form of
an injection. Most physicians choose to treat their patients with pills or skin patches. There are really no major
differences in the benefits regardless of the route of ad-
ministration. When estrogen is absorbed through a skin
patch, it gets into the circulation without first having to
be absorbed in the intestine and passing through the liver.

Estrogen can effectively relieve hot flashes, night
sweats, vaginal dryness, difficulty sleeping, and mood

swings. These benefits may vary somewhat from woman to woman, but in general, it is possible to find an effective dose of estrogen.

If a woman has a malignancy, then estrogen can accelerate its growth. Therefore the presence of cancer is a contraindication to estrogen replacement therapy.

The findings of current studies vary as to whether or not estrogen causes breast cancer. Although birth control pills have been associated with an increased risk of phlebitis and blood clot formation, the lower estrogen doses in hormonal replacement do not carry a similar high risk. Some women will experience worsening of headaches while taking estrogen, whereas others find that their headaches lessen. Extreme caution must be used when prescribing estrogen for women with active liver disease.

Progesterone, the other principal female hormone, is prescribed along with estrogen when a woman has a uterus. If she has had a hysterectomy and the uterus is absent, progesterone is not required, because its benefit is to reduce the risk of cancer of the uterus, which estrogen increases.

Progesterone has few side effects, but occasionally a woman will feel much more moody and depressed when taking it. The dose can usually be altered to alleviate this effect. However, some women just do not tolerate hormones well at all.

Estrogen and progesterone may be given in a cyclical manner (twenty-five to thirty days of estrogen and ten to twelve days of progesterone each month), and the woman will have a period each month. The two hormones can be given simultaneously, and those women will eventually stop having periods, although they may spot for quite a while before periods cease. Bleeding while taking estrogen should be considered abnormal and must be checked if it is not at the appropriate time each month.

A frequent question of menopausal women is, "How long do I have to take hormones?" The answer is, "As long as you are willing to take them." Why? Because the two major benefits of hormonal replacement are the prevention of osteoporosis and of heart attack, and these are lifelong risks after the ovaries stop producing normal amounts of estrogen. If, however, you have a history of breast, ovarian, or uterine cancer I would not recommend estrogen replacement therapy.

The manner in which estrogen works to prevent these severe problems is very technical, but I will describe it for you in simple terms.

Bones are made up of an interlacing network of calcium-laden material called the bony matrix. Calcium moves in and out of these areas to keep them strong. Weight bearing, that is, being on your feet and moving, and estrogen are necessary to keep calcium in the bone, otherwise the calcium moves out and the bone weakens. The end result of osteoporosis is "soft bones" and a greatly increased risk of fractures.

The arteries can slowly be lined with a substance called atherosclerotic plaque, which is primarily cholesterol. Men have higher rates of atherosclerotic change before midlife, but after menopause some women begin to develop atherosclerosis more rapidly. This laying down of plaque narrows the artery and can result in heart attacks and strokes. Estrogen acts directly on the arterial wall to decrease atherosclerosis. Therefore, estrogen helps to lower the rate of fatal heart attack in menopausal women.

Barbara read informational booklets and watched a videotape that I have done on menopause. She carefully considered the benefits and risks. Her mother, maternal grandmother, and two maternal aunts had severe osteoporosis, and she did not want to develop the same problem. She decided to start on a cyclical dose of oral estrogen and progesterone.

Occasionally a woman will consider the risks and decide not to take hormones. In that case, I encourage her to have a bone density test every two or three years and I give her medication to help her sleep if night sweats and difficulty sleeping are problems.

The menstrual cycle is marvelously intricate. Most women would prefer not to have bleeding and possibly cramping every month, but God has designed an intricate system to allow for regular preparation of the uterus for implantation of a fertilized egg.

Remember the close relationship between stress and periods. Controlling or relieving the stressors in your life can play a significant role in keeping your periods normal.

A Spiritual Perspective

Every woman is a unique display of the quality and nature of the female sex. This individual expression is a teacher to the generation of little girls who are watching and waiting to become women. I grew up in a family of women. My mother had three sisters, and I had an older sister. My father traveled all of my life, and we three "girls" (my mother, my sister, and I) spent a lot of time with Mother's sister in Mississippi. Though my aunts were married, my uncles do not predominate in my memories of girlhood. No, it was the strength of the female personalities that influenced me most. I believe our attitudes toward the challenges of living in a female body play a crucial role in the management of our physical health. I would like to suggest that you spend some time thinking about the manner in which you received your sex education. What emotions, if any, were attached to this information as it was conveyed to you?

Let me illustrate with a personal story.

One of my aunts was a nurse. Whenever we visited her house, my sister and I would surreptitiously retrieve dusty old obstetrical textbooks from the shelves. Since we were taught that matters of human reproduction and sexuality were for adults only, a sense of clandestine adventure drew us to the yellowed pages of these texts. As we perused the graphic illustrations of dilated cervixes and emerging fetuses, we were transfixed with wonder and horror in equal proportions. The seeds of my subsequent fears about pregnancy and childbirth were planted in those furtive moments. My sister and I heard our mother and her sisters tell gruesome tales of painful childbirth experiences, particularly the circumstances of our births, and these tales also left their marks on our psyches. Some of my girlfriends were initiated into the beginning of their menstrual cycles with phobic tales of pain and grim predictions of suffering to come. Mothers today have a great deal more information available to them and should be more savvy in their approach to female sex education.

My goal in this discussion is to point the reader toward a joyful acceptance of all that it means to be a woman created in the image of God. When we embrace the blessings as well as the challenges inherent in our sexual identity, we are moving in the direction of the healthy self-love the Bible speaks of when it commands us to love our neighbor the way we love ourselves (Mark 12:31). From the onset of the menstrual cycle through menopause and beyond, we will be given the opportunity to look on being female with gratitude or griping. My purpose is to exalt femininity, not above masculinity, but in a category all its own. I also exult in the creation of the male sex, and I praise God for men as equal expressions of the image of the divine.

In my lifetime, which began in 1949, I have witnessed an evolution in the definition of the term *feminine*. Common agreement on what it means to be female is no longer the norm. The bottom-line question is this: What does it mean to be a person who is created in the image of God? How does my perception of God affect my perception of myself and the living out of all that encompasses being a woman?

Let's look at our reflection of God's image. As long as we understand that the nature of God in its fullness encompasses all that it means to be male and female, I see no conflict nor any exclusivity at play in continuing to use the masculine pronoun in all references to our transcendent Creator. The stamp of the divine in me is simple; it is love. This divine love is the great equalizer—men are as capable of expression of divine love as women, as Jesus Christ demonstrated.

The energy of society in the nineties focuses on the pursuit of equality, but the standards of contemporary society can never be the norm for the Christian. The focus of our energy should be less on equality and more on the unraveling of the specific purposes assigned to us by our loving Creator for our brief time on this planet. There is deep purpose, protection, and provision for every phase of our lives, but that purpose is being focused on now. As we move from phase to phase, let that "nowness" be in our minds. There is deep joy available to us in the present but we cannot receive it with our minds fixed on the past or longing for the future.

Scriptures for Meditation

Ecclesiastes 7:10–12

Where and to whom will you look for ultimate wisdom? Does the Word of God hold the place of highest authority for you as you look for knowledge and insight?

Isaiah 43:1–3

As you move into uncharted territories in your interior and exterior life, consider the promise of God for his children stated in this passage of Isaiah. Do the promises of God apply to all generations or were they just for a special time and a particular people?

Jeremiah 6:16; 7:23

Do you consider the ancient words of God revealed in the Old Testament relevant for you and your circumstances today?

Daniel 2:22

Will you trust God's unconditional love enough to allow his light to penetrate even the dark hidden places of your inner person? Will you trust his wisdom above the wisdom of the world?

Suggested Spiritual Exercise

Perhaps it has never occurred to you to talk to the Lord about the way you acquired the sex education information you brought into adulthood. If it seems irrelevant to you now, simply read the suggested passages and construct your own exercise. If, however, you discover that you have come to the place you are in now with some wrong teaching that has hurt you or left you fearful, speak openly and honestly with the Lord concerning these matters. Ask him to show you the hidden places where you are in need of healing or new teaching. Thank him for the gift of being female. Ask him how you may use this gift for his glory.

5

Headaches

On a steamy, hot day in August, I rushed from the hospital to my office to start seeing my morning schedule of patients. I had finished a long surgical case, and I was running thirty minutes late. The patients and my staff would be anxiously awaiting my arrival. August is always very hot and very humid in central Kentucky, and today was no exception. Just as the car's air conditioner had begun to make an impact on the suffocating heat, I pulled into the office parking lot.

As I entered the back door to my consultation office, my nurse met me with a panicked look on her face.

"You've got to help us quickly," she said. "Beverly McAdams has a horrible headache and is just beside herself."

In the background, I heard a patient in the nearby exam room sobbing hysterically.

Beverly, a long-standing patient of mine, comes in annually for her physical examination, Pap smear, mammograms, and so forth, but frequently has to be seen for one or another of stress-related problems including irritable bowel syndrome, dysfunctional uterine bleeding, ulcer-related symptoms, and headaches. I had seen Beverly in some difficult situations before, but never had she seemed so distraught and in so much pain.

I quickly grabbed my lab coat, hooked a stethoscope around my neck, and headed for the room from which the cries emerged. As I opened the door, Beverly blurted out between sobs, "Oh, Dr. Hager, thank God you're here. Roger and his secretary—bad accident. I was at work. What am I going to do?"

"Beverly," I said, "stop, take a deep breath, and try to get hold of yourself. I cannot understand what you are trying to say." Beverly sobbed for another minute or so as I held her hands. Slowly she was able to regain her composure, and as she did, she began to complain of a severe pain in the right side of her head.

"Please turn the lights down," she pleaded. "My eyes hurt when they are on."

"Now," I interjected soothingly, "let's start from the beginning, and I'll try to help you." Painfully, Beverly began to relate her incredible story to my nurse and me. It seems that Roger, Beverly's husband, had lost his job recently and had felt quite depressed.

"While I was at work yesterday, Roger went out to the club to have some drinks. He called his former secretary, whom he had an affair with once, and took her with him. The police called and told me that Roger was in the emergency room, with lacerations on his head, cracked ribs, and a broken arm as a result of an accident. He had run a red light and hit another car broadside. His secretary wasn't injured."

Anger began to replace the sorrow in her voice. "I just don't know what I'm going to do," she stated.

Beverly is a very high-strung, emotional woman who has never resolved the stress in her life or modified it so that she would not suffer its physical consequences. Seeing her with stress-related symptoms was not unusual, but seeing her so severely symptomatic was alarming.

The emotional effect Roger's fling and accident had on Beverly was so powerful that it enabled her to distract herself from the severe pain of a migraine headache to relate the details to me. Once I was informed, however, her attention was drawn back to the pain in her head and neck.

Beverly has a long history of migraine headaches. They started when she was in college, and like most migraine sufferers, her headaches have manifested the same symptoms with each occurrence. Stress is usually the precipitating factor, but cured meats such as hot dogs and salami, pickled herring, and monosodium glutamate can also trigger an attack.

This migraine was characterized by a very sudden onset of severe, throbbing pain on both sides of the head, above the ears and behind the eyes, severe nausea and vomiting, sensitivity to light, sensitivity of the scalp to touch, and weakness. She was whimpering and holding her head again as the throbbing pain began to increase in intensity. Her color was ashen, and she had a glazed look in her eyes.

Fortunately, Beverly kept ergotamine in her purse, a medication used frequently in the treatment of migraines. We dimmed the lights, placed an ice pack on her head, and gave her a dose of the medication. Within twenty minutes the pain was beginning to subside, and Beverly said to my nurse, Lisa, "I want to get up and go home."

We did not want Beverly to drive, since recurrence of these severe symptoms was possible. I phoned her sister and asked her to come and take Beverly home with her, away from Roger. I knew that Beverly still had to face an injured, unfaithful husband and that she did not need that major confrontation now.

The Impact of Headaches

Doesn't everybody have headaches? They come and they go. It's just something that we have to learn to live with. So why do we even bother discussing such a common problem?

Headaches are another stress-related disorder, and by learning to resolve stress, we can have an impact on their frequency and severity. Remember, we do not have to be victimized by stress and suffer its consequences.

Headaches are the ninth leading cause of visits to doctors' offices. They are a major cause of pain and disability, resulting in frequent days off from work and significant financial loss for individuals and for companies. Seldom a day goes by that I don't see someone in the office with headache as a major complaint.

We even call a certain type of headache a "tension headache." Though stress may trigger all of the various types of headaches, not all headaches are tension headaches. The table that follows lists the principal types of headaches occurring in women, with their common symptoms and precipitating factors. Women, more frequently than men, suffer headaches.

Headaches and Their Symptoms

Four kinds of stress-related headaches can be identified and differentiated by their symptoms. Migraine headaches are divided into two major categories, classic and common migraines. In addition, there are cluster headaches, which occur principally in men, and menstrual migraines, which are a variant of the common migraine but occur only in association with a woman's periods.

Stress results in the release of hormones such as serotonin and histamine into the blood stream. These hormones can result in vascular spasm—intermittent narrowing of blood vessels—which causes pain. It was formerly taught that migraine headaches were "vascular headaches," resulting from this narrowing of blood vessels, and that tension headaches did not involve vascular spasm. We now know that both types of headache can involve relaxation or widening of blood vessels, and this is why stress can play a role in causing all types of headaches.

Types of Headaches in Women

Type	Location	Symptoms	Precipitating Factors
Classic migraine	Usually one side of head (front, back, or sides)	Preceded by aura of neurologic symptoms, throbbing pain, nausea, vomiting, weakness, sensitivity to noise or light, numbness of hands or mouth, blindness, weakness of limbs, inability to speak, dizziness, lights before eyes	Mood changes, stress, bright lights, alcohol, certain foods
Common migraine	Frequently bilateral (front, back, or sides of head; behind eyes)	Not preceded by an aura; throbbing pain, nausea and vomiting, weakness, sensitive scalp	Bright lights, noise, stress, alcohol, certain foods
Tension headache	Over entire head and often neck and shoulders	Viselike tightness and pain	Fear, worry, anxiety, depression
Menstrual migraine	May be localized or generalized	Throbbing pain, nausea, vomiting, weakness	Always associated with menses and stress

Classic Migraines

Usually located in the front or back, on one side of the head, classic migraines are always preceded by what is called an "aura"—one or several symptoms that always occur just before the headache begins. These may include neurologic symptoms like bright lights dancing before the eyes, blindness or a partial cut in the field of vision, numbness in the hands or mouth, weakness in the extremities or in the mouth, inability to speak, and dizziness. The headache is sudden in onset, throbbing in nature, and almost always associated with nausea and/or vomiting, weakness, and sensitivity to light and noise.

The headache may last from a few hours to two or three days. Although stress is often a precipitating factor, sudden mood changes, bright lights, loud noises, alcohol, and certain foods may precede the event. Darkness, sleep, and specific medications help relieve the symptoms.

Common Migraines

Common migraines are more frequent than classic migraine headaches. They are usually located in the front of the head or on the sides, in the temple area. The major distinguishing factor between classic and common migraines is that common migraines do not have an aura before the headache begins. The pain is usually sudden in onset and throbbing in nature. After a period of time, the pain may dissipate, becoming a generalized, dull ache. Common migraines are frequently associated with nausea and vomiting. The scalp may become sensitive to the touch.

These headaches may occur anytime during the day; sometimes they are even present upon awakening in the morning. They last anywhere from a few hours to one or two days.

Tension and stress, bright lights, loud noises, and alcohol may precipitate a common migraine headache. There are usually no specific neurologic symptoms like those described with classic migraines. Darkness, sleep, and medication may also effectively treat common migraines, but reduction of stress is the best prevention.

Tension Headaches

These are characterized by a steady, nonpulsatile aching, which may originate in any area of the head. Tension headaches usually move to the front or back of the head but are often on both sides of those areas and make the sufferer feel as if she has a tight band around her head. These headaches are frequently termed muscle-contraction headaches, because the muscles in the head and the neck become very sore. These headaches may be just as severe as migraines. Dizziness and blurred vision may occur, but nausea, vomiting, weakness, and specific neurologic symptoms do not. As the name would suggest, these headaches result from tension, anxiety, depression, and sometimes from a posture that causes muscle contractions and eventually spasm. Theoretically, spasm may result in an accumulation of substances in muscles that sensitizes the nerve endings to pain.

Like migraines, tension headaches are definitely more frequent in women. They often occur late in the afternoon or at night—after a stressful day. They may persist for days or even months.

Rest and stress resolution are the best modes of treatment for tension headaches. Though medication may relieve the symptoms, it does not resolve the underlying cause.

Menstrual Migraines

Menstrual migraines are characterized by the same symptoms and location as common migraines, but the onset of headaches is always associated with a menstrual period. The pain usually resolves with the end of a period. Medications that counteract the effects of prostaglandins (any of a group of powerful substances with hormonelike effects) in the body frequently provide effective treatment. An example of this type of medication is ibuprofen.

Carol has never seemed to be a happy, contented person. I remember the first time I saw her, on a beautiful spring day when the sun had begun to reappear after taking a winter-long vacation. The tulips and crocuses were blooming, and everyone seemed alive with spring fever.

Everyone, that is, except Carol.

She was in my office for an examination. I walked into the exam room and was greeted by a very attractive, small, blond woman who had a scowl on her face that would make you gasp. As a matter of fact, I recall that I did just that. I introduced myself, and Carol replied, "I really don't feel well. I have a headache, my back is really hurting, my stomach hurts right here," she continued, pointing to her left groin. "My hip hurts, and I haven't been sleeping well."

It turned out that tax season had taken its toll on Carol, an accountant, and, as frequently occurred, her body was feeling much of her tension and anxiety. However, her severe migraine headaches seemed to be her major problem. I asked her to describe her symptoms. From her description, I could have written a book on classic migraines.

"Whenever I get tired or am under a lot of stress at work or at home, I develop a headache. My mother and sister have the same kind of headaches. I get these bright orange lights in my eyes, and I hear a very high-pitched sound. I know it's coming then. Very quickly, I begin to get weak, I get nauseated, and vomit. I get numb on the left side of my face and feel tingling in my arm. Light and noise make my headaches much worse. Sometimes I can't see out of my left eye. I have to get in the dark and lie down with a cold rag on my head, or I might pass out."

I found out that Carol had been diagnosed by a neurologist as having classic migraine disorder. She was supposed to be taking a daily dose of propranolol—medication to control the frequency of her headaches—but she often forgot it.

Carol had a very difficult marriage to a man who was not sympathetic toward her maladies. He was addicted to alcohol and had difficulty holding a job. She had low self-esteem and seemingly had no joy in her life at all.

I tried to outline a strategy for Carol that would involve stress reduction and counseling, but she said, "I don't have time for counseling. I'm not crazy, and I just need medication to relieve my headache."

She didn't have time to take her propranolol every day, so she wanted a quick fix to relieve this headache, ignoring the fact that another one could occur at any time.

Carol was an unfortunate victim of a familial disorder—migraine disease. Although she could not change the circumstances of her birth (Carol's mother and grandmother both had migraine disease), Carol could take steps to alter the stress in her life, since stress and tension frequently precipitated her headaches.

It isn't easy to reduce stress, but when you know that it is contributing to disease in your life, it is necessary to make changes.

Many people find that migraine headaches are precipitated by events or substances. Avoiding those can reduce the frequency of headaches. Staying away from bright or flashing lights and loud noises is important. Some dietary suggestions for migraine sufferers are listed in the following table.

In spite of the best preventive efforts, some women will fall victim to migraine headaches. The key is to find a medication that works for the specific patient. If the headaches do not resolve, or they are not typical, an electroencephalogram (EEG) and/or a magnetic resonance imaging (MRI) of the head may be in order to rule out a possible tumor.

Dietary Suggestions for Migraine Sufferers

Avoid alcohol, especially red wines and champagnes.
Avoid strong or aged cheeses.
Avoid chicken livers, pickled herring, canned figs, and pods of broad beans.
Use monosodium glutamate sparingly.
Avoid cured meats such as hot dogs, bacon, or salami if they cause headaches.
Eat three balanced meals a day.
Avoid fasting.

Connie came to see me, convinced that she was having headaches because her "hormones were messed up."

Connie is a twenty-nine-year-old nurse in the surgical intensive care unit at a local hospital. She has two young children at home. Her husband, a computer programmer, attends night school, working to earn a master's degree. Her youngest son has many problems with allergies.

She described headaches that were persistent and getting progressively worse. The pain she described was like a tight band around her head. It was constant and often extended to her neck and shoulders, which ached and spasmed. The headaches would get worse at work and often lasted for days without remission.

I treated Connie with medication, but she experienced only partial relief of her headaches. At that point, I suggested that she ask her supervisor for a transfer to a less stressful unit. I also talked with her husband about helping Connie with the household duties. Those two changes made the difference in recovery from these debilitating headaches. Slowly they began to decrease in intensity and then in duration. She is enjoying life much more now that her stress level is lower.

If, like Connie, you have tension headaches, what can you do to help yourself? You must take steps to decrease the tension resulting from stress. Consider taking time for relaxation at work and for a few minutes when you first get home. Get involved in an exercise program to help reduce stress and to release natural pain relievers into your bloodstream. Avoid alcohol, caffeine, and nicotine. (If you are addicted to any of these, you must slowly decrease your consumption. When I quit caffeine cold turkey, I had severe headaches for several weeks. Try to avoid taking excessive amounts of aspirin or acetaminophen for pain relief.) Begin a dedicated time for meditation, prayer, and spiritual growth. You will be amazed at the calming effect that these times can have.

Talk to someone. Your spouse, boyfriend, close friend, or counselor can be a valuable aid in helping to dissipate your stress. Help your husband or boyfriend to understand how you feel. Remember that men do not have headaches as frequently as women, and the man in your life may not comprehend what you are going through. Get your feelings out and deal with them. You will find that you can conquer stress and have an impact on its effects.

Remember, we all have stresses but we do not have to let them control our lives and inflict us with disease.

> In all these things we overwhelmingly conquer through Him who loved us.
>
> Romans 8:37

A Spiritual Perspective

Have you heard that saying, "Pain is inevitable; misery is optional"? Obviously, this implies that we have a choice in terms of our response to the suffering that comes across our paths during our journeys through life.

Beverly and Carol are fictitious patients, but their cases are a composite of many similar cases David sees weekly in his practice. We could spend a great deal of time talking about the way the choices their mates have made have contributed to the physical pain these women are suffering. But if they concentrate their energies on laying blame, they will miss the treasure hidden in the field of their suffering.

"Treasure?" you say.

Oh, yes, my friend. As you lie in a darkened room, drifting through thin layers of consciousness, waiting for the medicine to take away your pain, there is a treasure waiting to be uncovered—newfound intimacy with the God of the universe, through the power of his Holy Spirit. Beverly and Carol, as well as their mates, are suffering from the unmet need for true intimacy that is the universal heart cry of humanity. How often that treasured intimacy is hidden in a field of suffering.

In his classic work, *Prayer,* O. Hallesby teaches us "how graciously prayer has been designed.

"To pray is nothing more involved than to let Jesus into our need. To pray is to give Jesus permission to employ His powers in the alleviation of our distress. Will we give Jesus access to our needs?" Hallesby tells us that this is "the one great fundamental question in connection with prayer. Prayer is an attitude of our hearts, an attitude of mind toward God, an attitude which He in heaven immediately recognizes as prayer, as an appeal to His heart. Whether it takes the form of words or not, does not mean anything to God, only to ourselves." Hallesby goes on to say: "The only necessary spiritual condition of prayer is helplessness. Our helplessness is a continual appeal to His father-heart."[1]

Wherever you are in your journey, I want to encourage you to take this present moment to turn your heart toward the heart of the Father and to invite him into your pain. In biblical language, Jesus calls this act of entering in to "sup with us." The common meal is symbolic of intimate and joyous fellowship. Hallesby says: "This affords a new glimpse into the nature of prayer, showing us that God has designed prayer as a means of intimate and joyous fellowship between God and humankind."[2] Our heads will begin to cease aching as our hearts begin their breaking under the gentle touch of our Father's hand.

Scriptures for Meditation

Matthew 13:44–46

Imagine yourself traveling down one of the winding back roads of your state. It is a hot, humid summer afternoon. You're looking for a place to stop and rest for a while. Finally you pull off the road near an open field. A few ancient oaks line an overgrown lane leading to someone's farm. You stop under them to rest in the shade of their spreading branches. As you are resting, an old man approaches your car. He looks harmless enough so you lean out the window of your car to speak to him.

He beats you to the punch, calling out as he comes near, "You must be another one of those people lookin' to bury this field."

What would anyone want with this dried up, deserted piece of property in the middle of nowhere? you ask yourself, but reply: "No sir, I'm just stopping to rest for a bit. Hope you don't mind. I mean, if this is your place, I hope it's okay for me to pull off the shoulder here. These shade trees are so inviting."

"Don't make me no never mind," the old man replies. "This is my land all right. Us Hoffmans have farmed it for a long time. But I'm lookin' to sell it. There's folks say there could be oil out here, but I ain't got the wherewithal to go lookin' for it. I figure if there's oil it would've sprung up a long time ago, with all the plowin' we've done over the years."

You nod, agreeing that nothing valuable could be found in this old barren field. "You're probably right, but with what you could sell it for, you could take it easy for the rest of your life."

"Umph," the old man snorts. "Ain't lookin' to make a killin' off it. I just want what's fair. I've got fifty acres here. I'm sellin' it for ten thousand dollars."

You smile, say good-bye, and head for home. A few weeks pass. You've forgotten your rest stop and the conversation with the old farmer. As you sit in a carpool line one afternoon you turn on the radio. The deejay on your favorite station is commenting on the news.

"Seems that an old fellow by the name of Arvel Elmo Hoffman has become a multimillionaire! Oil has been found on the property that has been in the Hoffman family for generations. Hoffman says the land never was that good for farming but he's glad he hung on to it. You just never know what's hidden out in those fields!"

Reread Matthew 13:44–46. Like Mr. Hoffman's empty, unexplored fields, there are vast, unexplored areas within our spiritual selves. There are spiritual treasures hidden in those interior "lands" of which we may never be aware. Why? Because the price of spiritual prospecting is often too high.

For the last twenty-eight years the Holy Spirit has been my guide in the exploration of my own interior lands. Our journey has led me up into the high places and carried me across deep valleys. I know the thirst and the loneliness of the dry desert places as well as the peace of the still pastureland. My adventure has involved laying aside my own desires and my own ways of finding the promised land. I am still learning to discipline myself to work hard, to be open to the correction of the Lord of the land, and to be content with delayed gratification rather than the immediate rewards I desire. But oh, my friend, as the fields of suffering have offered up their treasures I have come into priceless spiritual wealth.

Would you be willing to embrace the suffering you are now experiencing if you believed the suffering could be redeemed, becoming blessing and wholeness?

Revelation 3:17–22

What is the counsel of the Lord in this passage? How can you apply this counsel to the pressure and tension you are facing?

What is the promised response of the Lord to those who invite him to enter into their circumstances?

Song of Solomon 2

Feast on these words and then try the suggested spiritual exercise.

Suggested Spiritual Exercise

Spread a soft quilt over your bed. Lie down with a comfortable pillow under your head and another under your knees. If need be, cover up with a warm blanket or smooth sheet. Close your eyes and become aware of the pattern of your breathing. Lose yourself in the soft grayness of the natural daylight or the enveloping darkness of evening.

Now imagine that Jesus has come into the room and is sitting in a chair beside your bed. He is asking nothing of you. No words are necessary as you commune heart to heart. The silence between the two of you is comforting and reassuring. Receive his presence and imagine the light and love that emanate from him, touching you at the point of your deepest pain. Remember the words of Song of Songs 2:3 (NIV): "I delight to sit in his shade, and his fruit is sweet to my taste. He has taken me to the banquet hall and his banner over me is love."

6

Irritable Bowel Syndrome

The sudden, sharp ringing startled me out of sleep. As I reached for the phone I struggled to get the cobwebs out of my head and determine where I was.

"Dr. Hager, we have Charlotte Kendall here in the emergency room, complaining of severe abdominal pain. You know she has been here several times before with similar problems. She is requesting that you see her," said the voice on the other end of the line.

I had been at the hospital most of the night. At 4:00 A.M. I arrived home and fell into a deep sleep. Now, forty-five minutes later, it was a struggle to remember who I was, much less who Charlotte Kendall was. As the emergency room nurse spoke, the detailed and complicated history of this young woman began to play through my mind.

Charlotte is a beautiful young woman who is employed as a receptionist by a busy real estate firm. Her life has been beset by one difficult situation after another. Raised by her mother after her father left home when she was twelve years old, Charlotte had low self-esteem. She was very bright and did well in school. Her beauty enabled her to be popular and accepted by the in crowd in high school. She dated extensively, but she could never establish a lasting relationship.

Near the end of her senior year, Charlotte found out that she was pregnant. The father of the child refused to accept any responsibility, and she decided that the only option open to her was to have an abortion. After the abortion, she became extremely depressed. In order to escape the whispers and gossip of family and friends, she moved to Lexington to get a job and attend night school.

Unfortunately, she found employment with a real estate firm whose unscrupulous owner recognized a vulnerable young woman when he saw one. The requests to stay late and do extra work and to do special favors for the boss quickly ensued. Opportunities for advancement and pay raises were tied to her cooperation with his sexual demands. Because she wanted to be accepted and loved, Charlotte acquiesced. She felt guilty but did not tell anyone about her activities.

She had never taken good care of herself physically. While in high school, her diet was typical of most young people—junk food. In order to maintain what she perceived was an ideal weight, she would frequently purge. Binge eating to defuse tension and anxiety was commonplace. Frequent colds and flu typified her medical history. Aspirin for headaches and diet pills for weight reduction were the mainstays of her medicine chest.

I saw Charlotte in the office for the first time four years ago with complaints of abdominal pain and episodes of diarrhea. She had been seen by another physician the year before and had been treated twice with antibiotics for pelvic inflammatory disease (PID), an infection of the fallopian tubes that causes abdominal and pelvic pain. She came to see me because she was frustrated that the infections were recurring.

"I just can't relax," she said. "It seems that everything I do, everything that happens to me, results in more stress. I have to go to school, to do what I have to at work, and if I refuse my boss's overtures, I could lose my job. I keep having one episode of pain after another."

I asked her to describe the nature of her pain, realizing that I was also going to have to deal with her serious emotional issues before she left the office that day.

"The pain comes unexpectedly," Charlotte related. "It starts as a dull ache and then suddenly I have severe pain in my lower abdomen. I feel bloated and usually have diarrhea. It may last for a few hours or even a few days."

"Is the pain usually on both sides?" I asked.

"No, it is usually worse on the left and may not hurt on the right at all."

"Do you ever have fever, abnormal vaginal discharge, or abnormal bleeding?"

"No, never," the young woman answered.

Charlotte's examination revealed nothing out of the ordinary, physically. Her abdominal exam was unremarkable, and her pelvic examination revealed no abnormal masses and only slight tenderness in the area of the left ovary and sigmoid colon (the portion of the large bowel that leads to the rectum). A microscopic evaluation of vaginal secretions revealed no increase in white blood cells, bacteria, or yeast. It seemed obvious that Charlotte did not have PID and probably had a disorder known as irritable bowel syndrome (IBS).

I told her that reduction of stress was key to her treatment. I advised her in appropriate dietary change, fluid intake, and exercise. I prescribed a medication to use, should the abdominal cramping become severe.

"Charlotte," I said, "you must get out of your current job situation before it destroys you." I referred her to the appropriate authorities to report the sexual harassment and gave her the names of two singles' groups at local churches. I emphasized to her that spiritual wholeness would pave the way to emotional and physical wholeness.

Now the emergency room nurse was waiting for my answer. "I will be there in just a few minutes," I told her over the phone. I quickly dressed to return to the hospital.

Charlotte had not heeded the advice I'd given. She remained at the real estate firm, in an addictive manner allowing the harassment to continue. She made no changes in her diet and continued to avoid exercise.

In the meantime, she had seen another gynecologist who laparoscoped her for chronic abdominal and pelvic pain (laparoscopy is a surgical procedure where a lighted instrument is introduced into the abdomen through the navel, so that the abdominal and pelvic organs can be seen). He told her that she had a small cyst of the right ovary and drained the fluid from it. She had also been seen at an outpatient treatment center and again received antibiotics for PID without having any definite diagnosis.

She had returned to my care two years before this emergency room visit. Her emotional state was chaotic, and she continued having episodes of abdominal pain, back pain, and tension-type headaches. She denied any recent behavior consistent with anorexia. Due to the worsening severity of her pain and her insistence that there had to be something organically wrong, I scheduled her for repeat laparoscopy. This revealed no abnormal findings in the pelvis, except for a rather large, redundant colon, which may be seen in patients with irritable bowel syndrome.

Once again, she had been given the advice to change her work environment, get into counseling, and change her diet. Tonight she was back in the emergency room with the same symptoms, requesting narcotics to relieve the pain.

I parked in the physicians' parking lot and walked through the emergency department entrance.

"She's in room 10, Dr. Hager," the clerk stated. I picked up her chart and walked into the examination room.

"Please don't be upset with me," Charlotte blurted. "But the pain is so bad you have to do something to help me."

"Charlotte, I'll be happy to examine you, but if your findings haven't changed, I'm going to insist that you follow through with my previous advice, or I won't see you again, because I can't help you."

The examination was no different than before. The pain was severe and on the left side of her abdomen. All her laboratory values from the blood that had been drawn were normal.

"I will give you a prescription to help with the bowel spasm, but you do not need narcotics."

As she began to cry, she whispered, "I know you're right. Please refer me to a counselor so that I can get the help I need. I can't go on like this."

Finally, Charlotte was at such a low point that the emotional as well as the physical pain brought her to the brink of desperation. Aware that she had to have help from outside herself, she got into counseling with a Christian psychologist. Slowly she was able to change her diet to include more fiber and less greasy food. She initiated a regular exercise program. She also began to attend a local church regularly. You wouldn't recognize Charlotte as the same forlorn woman who sat sobbing in a hospital emergency room. She is bright, energetic, vivacious and is making a difference in her community.

Chronic Bowel Dysfunction

The physical and emotional consequences of stress are devastating, yet until the pain gets severe enough, most people are not willing to make the changes necessary to resolve their stress-related diseases.

I don't want you to wait until you have symptoms of stress-related disorders before you take steps to resolve your stress. Each year in the United States, over thirty million persons suffer from acute or chronic digestive dysfunction. Diseases that are included in this list of diagnoses are inflammatory bowel disease, such as Crohn's disease and ulcerative colitis; diverticular disease of the colon, which can be complicated by infection (diverticulitis); and irritable bowel syndrome, one of the stress-related disorders that we see frequently among women.

Bowel function is affected by many things. As children, the type of diet we eat and the bowel habits we develop play a critical role in the way our bowels function later in life. In Africa, for example, where children eat diets high in fiber, their colons are stretched by the fiber content and are rather large. The incidence of digestive disorders later in life is low.

Frequently, children are hesitant to have bowel movements when away from home. At school they hold things in. As a result, the individual does not learn to respond to the natural after-meal impulse to empty the colon, and constipation or bowel spasm can result. Increasing fiber in the diet, when this has not been done before, can distend—swell—the colon and actually result in more bowel spasm and pain. It is important to teach our children to eat adequate fiber diets with low fat content, but not excessive fiber.

Irritable bowel syndrome is one of the most frequently diagnosed digestive disorders. It should not be a "wastebasket diagnosis," made only when we cannot figure out anything else to call the problem. Patients with IBS will have crampy abdominal pain, either diarrhea or constipation, frequently hyperactive bowel sounds (groaning and churning of the intestines), and no other obvious cause for pain.

The pain associated with IBS is often relieved by the passage of stool or gas. There is often a strong sense of urgency before the passage of loose or watery stools. When diarrhea is present, it is usually associated with meals and frequently occurs early in the day. Constipation can be either the passage of small quantities of stool or infrequent bowel movements. Gas can present a tight, bloated sensation, belching, or excessive flatus (gas released through the rectum). Symptoms are intermingled so that they are usually unique to the particular person.

Bowel habits in women with IBS are usually irregular. A week of constipation followed by several days of diarrhea is not unusual. Nausea and altered appetite may occur. Some patients notice an increased amount of mucus in their stools. There is almost always some over-lying emotional component to the history, with major de-grees of stress involved.

Not everyone is like Charlotte. You may only have symp-toms when you are maximally stressed. Perhaps in the midst of a hectic day you are racing through the mall, and sud-denly you feel that something inside has grabbed your in-testines and is squeezing them. You struggle to make it to the rest room for the first of several bouts of diarrhea. By the next day, you are more relaxed, and the symptoms abate.

Studies have shown that persons with IBS have a stronger reaction to stress than do individuals who have abdominal pain but do not meet the other diagnostic cri-teria for IBS. Patients with IBS were studied under hypno-sis. Hypnotically inducing the emotions of excitement and anger worsened symptoms, whereas inducing the emotion of happiness lessened symptoms. Stress has been shown to increase movement and spasm in the colon (large in-testine) but to have no such effect on the small intestine.

IBS is a diagnosis of exclusion. In other words, other dis-orders must be ruled out before the diagnosis can be made. PID, ovarian cysts, endometriosis, severe hemorrhoids, in-flammatory bowel disease, and polyps of the colon may present similar symptoms. Inflammatory bowel disease usually results in blood or pus in the stool. Colonoscopy—in which an instrument is inserted through the rectum in order to see the colon—is necessary to make this diagno-sis as well as to identify colonic polyps. Intolerance to milk, fructose, or wheat gluten not infrequently has the princi-pal symptoms of crampy abdominal pain and diarrhea. Parasitic infections such as giardiasis can occur as a result of drinking impure water. Diarrhea and cramping are the usual symptoms. Cancer of the colon usually presents with pain or bleeding from the rectum. Loss of appetite and weight loss are seen in advanced disease.

The pain with IBS is quite migratory across the lower abdomen, but the focus is usually in the left lower quadrant. At laparoscopy, we have noted that these women tend to have a rather large colon with increased folding, or redundancy. There are no other specific findings when the bowel is seen. At colonoscopy, increased spasm may be noted.

The hormones released into the bloodstream when you are stressed cause many effects that have previously been mentioned. One such effect is increased contraction in the bowel resulting from spasm in the smooth muscle lining of the intestine. Spasm of any organ results in pain. The rapid contraction may prevent appropriate liquid absorption in the colon, and diarrhea results.

Constipation may also occur in women with IBS. Constipation is the most common gastrointestinal complaint in the United States, with 2.5 million persons visiting doctors' offices each year with this finding. Bowel movements occurring two to three times a week to two to three times a day can be considered normal. Constipation is defined as the infrequent and difficult passage of small amounts of hard stool. Causes of constipation associated with IBS, in addition to stress, may include inadequate fiber and/or fluid intake, medications such as narcotics that slow bowel function, pregnancy, and lack of exercise. Correcting these deficiencies is the best therapy, especially increasing fiber, exercise, and fluids. The latter factors are also key to the treatment of IBS. If you are experiencing the classic symptoms of this disorder, and other causes of abdominal and pelvic pain have been eliminated, there are steps that you can take to decrease your symptoms.

If you take appropriate action and your symptoms do not improve, a complete gastrointestinal evaluation should be performed.

There are certain foods that persons with IBS should avoid. Beans, nuts, cabbage, raisins, milk products including ice cream, mushrooms, and very spicy foods promote the production of gas and worsen the symptoms of bloating and cramping. You should find out if you have lactose intolerance, in which case you must avoid all milk products. You may find that eliminating chocolate and caffeine from your diet is beneficial.

Increasing the amount of fiber you eat is the most important aspect of management. Most Americans average ten to fifteen grams of fiber a day, women frequently less than that. Most nutritionists recommend twenty to thirty-five grams a day. The following table lists foods that have good fiber content. Beans are listed but should be eaten in limited amounts because of gas production. Corn and its related products should not be consumed if bowel spasm results from their intake.

Food Fiber Content

Food	Serving Size	Total Fiber (in grams)
Beans		
green/string beans	1/2 cup	1.89
brown beans	1/2 cup	4.64
red beans	1/2 cup	5.48
kidney beans	1/2 cup	5.48
lima beans	1/2 cup	4.25
navy beans	1/2 cup	7.72
Vegetables		
spinach	1/2 cup	2.07
broccoli	1/2 cup	2.58
carrots	1/2 cup	2.42
corn	1/2 cup	3.03

(continued)

(*Food Fiber Content—continued*)

Food	Serving Size	Total Fiber (in grams)
green peas	1/2 cup	3.36
potatoes (baked with skin)	1/2 cup	1.95
Fruits		
apple, with peel	1 medium	2.76
banana	1 medium	2.19
boysenberries	1 cup	7.20
cherries	1 cup	1.88
pear, with peel	1 medium	4.32
prunes, canned	1 cup	13.76
Breads		
whole wheat bread	1 slice	2.11
white bread	1 slice	.50
bran bread	1 slice	2.66
cornbread	1 medium piece	1.24
multigrain bread	1 slice	1.92
rye bread	1 slice	1.72
Grains/Cereals		
barley	1/2 cup	15.80
cornmeal	1/2 cup	3.59
whole wheat flour	1/2 cup	6.58
brown rice	1/2 cup	5.27
bran cereal	1 ounce	5.27
shredded wheat cereal	1 ounce	2.64

In addition to fiber, it is important to eat regular meals and chew your food thoroughly. You should drink six to eight glasses of fluid a day and exercise regularly (three or four days per week). Responding to the natural urge to empty your bowels is important so that you avoid straining later. There is a normal bodily reaction called the gastrocolic reflex that promotes emptying of the colon. When you eat, your stomach fills and the brain sends an impulse to the colon to empty, to allow for proper digestion and passage of the meal. Not responding to this reflex can result in increased gas production and constipation. Although all of the above are important, the elimination of stress is the key to avoiding problems with IBS. Stress-management programs have been shown to have a statistically significant benefit in decreasing IBS symptoms. Heed the advice given to Charlotte. Alter the stress at work by changing jobs or changing the environment you work in. If there are relational stresses with your spouse, your mother, your child, your employer, you should seek counseling. Change your lifestyle by eating a proper diet, drinking plenty of fluids, and exercising regularly. Stress-related disorders like IBS can be managed so your symptoms decrease.

> Casting all your anxiety on Him, because He cares for you. Be of sober spirit, be on the alert. Your adversary, the devil, prowls about like a roaring lion, seeking someone to devour.
>
> 1 Peter 5:7–8

A Spiritual Perspective

Does it ever seem to you that you are playing out your life to an audience that does not exist? Our case study, Charlotte, reminds me of such a person. The events that occur during the formative years of adolescence often continue to cast their shadows across our paths long after adolescence is past. We allow those people who may have criticized or rejected us for completely invalid and childish reasons to continue to be powerful influences in the choices we make, even though we may live many miles, even many states, away from the scene of our teen years. Eventually, as in Charlotte's case, our bodies will begin to show the stress we place upon ourselves to live up to an image or to run from our pain. For some of us, that bodily expression will take the form of IBS.

All through this book, I am attempting to help us gain a spiritual perspective on our physical problems. I do not believe that spiritualizing our pain can make it disappear. That would be dishonest, unscriptural, and a gross insult to the character of God. Rather, I am encouraging you to see physical pain as a red flag—a signal from your body that you should not ignore. Try to examine your pain from more than one perspective. Are the choices you are making the result of well thought out, prayerful contemplation, or do you live driven by the terrible tyranny of the "ought and should"? Do you pay the perpetual penance of regret?

When we hurt, the Creator-given innate wisdom of our bodies is seeking to teach us a better way, a way that takes account of the whole person. A wise physician will tell you that he or she may be able to cooperate with God in healing your physical pain, but that healing will be greatly hampered if the core issues of your inner person are not given the attention they deserve. I want to encourage you to move toward your pain. See it as a multidimensional entity. If we treat our bodies but fail to care for our souls, we will live half-lives, never touched by the abundance that Jesus is able and longing to bring to us.

Scriptures for Meditation

Romans 5:1–11

Is there any good that can come from suffering?

Matthew 10:28

When we become ill there is a sense of helplessness that leads to deep fear. It may be some time before we receive the proper diagnosis and/or treatment. Even when treatment begins we may have difficulty adjusting and tolerating the treatment. In such times it is a blessed thing to realize that while we cannot control what is happening to our bodies we *can* participate in the "soul care" that the Holy Spirit desires to bring to us. How does this verse in Matthew help you put your illness in perspective?

Deuteronomy 4:29–31

If you want to feel the nearness of the Lord, you must do something. Check verse 29 to see what is required of you.

What do these verses tell you about the nature and character of your heavenly Father? How will a father like this care for you when you are hurting?

Continually return to the Lord. If you slip away, return to the Lord.

Joshua 22:4–5

What do these verses tell us we must do to maintain our relationship with our heavenly Father? What should the attitude of our hearts be after God has moved on our behalf?

Psalm 6

Ancient people of biblical times suffered just as we suffer today. What is the hope that the psalmist clings to in his pain and suffering? Our God is his God.

Suggested Spiritual Exercise

Carve out a block of time when you can take yourself on a solitary retreat. If you are able to leave your home and go to a quiet place, removed from your usual circumstances, then do so. If the quietness of a room in your house is your only real choice, that will also suffice. The goal of this exercise is the experience of solitude. Dare to face yourself with fierce honesty and deliberate scrutiny. Be aware of the fact that God sees what is secret from others. He loves you just as you are, and he views your feeble frame with compassion. Remember the words of that ancient prayer that tell us: "Thou art the God whose property is ALWAYS to be MERCIFUL."[1] If, in the past, you have closed your mind to uncomfortable thoughts, make a conscious decision here in the presence of your Creator to be present to those things which make their home in your shadow-self. Invite the great Comforter, the Holy Spirit, to walk with you into the shadows. Imagine him taking your hand into his just now, and feel the way his perfect love is removing your worst fears. Now, covenant with him to begin to make your decisions in the light of this love and in the knowledge of his never ending mercy. Claim Philippians 3:13–16.

7

Fibromyalgia

*I*n my practice, I frequently see women with any one of a number of stress-related disorders. On any given day, I may see several patients with headaches, irritable bowel syndrome, menstrual disorders, or eating disorders, some with one problem, some with a combination of disorders. Recently, however, I have been seeing more and more women with rather severe joint and muscle pain, a constellation of symptoms known as fibromyalgia (formerly called fibrositis). This disorder is linked to a condition known as chronic fatigue syndrome.

Is it that I have finally learned enough about the disorder to diagnose it, or are there truly more cases occurring now? Many experts think that although fibromyalgia has been around for a long time (a similar condition is described in the Book of Job), the stresses of today's lifestyle have resulted in more cases occurring. In the United States, an estimated three to six million persons are afflicted, 80 percent of them women.

Barbara Daner is one of those women. The first time I saw Barbara she was attending a high school football game. I noticed her because she seemed to be so uncomfortable. She was walking in a sort of stooped manner, and her arms did not swing freely as she moved. There was a grimace on her face.

Much to my surprise, Barbara appeared in my office the following week as a gynecologic patient. She had made an appointment several weeks earlier. Barbara had no significant gynecologic complaints and was there for a routine checkup and Pap smear, but as her history unfolded, it was obvious that she had several problems that deserved attention.

"I have to be honest with you," Barbara admitted. "I am here out of desperation. I have been to several other physicians, and no one seems to know what is wrong with me."

She had an urgent tone in her voice as she explained, "I just thought that perhaps my symptoms might be related to my hormones, so I came here."

"Tell me what bothers you the most, Barbara," I urged.

"It's really hard to put into words," she stated. "Basically, I'm exhausted. I have a lot of pain from my irritable bowel, with diarrhea one day and constipation the next. The thing that bothers me the most, though, is the discomfort I have in my neck, shoulders, back, and hips."

I encouraged her to continue.

"About two years ago, I began to notice that I was very tired all the time," she stated. "I hadn't been this worn out since I had mononucleosis in high school. I found it difficult to get up in the morning. Because I was very stiff, I thought that I probably had arthritis, so I went to see my family physician. He examined me and didn't find anything unusual. Some lab tests were ordered, including a test for rheumatoid arthritis, and they all came back negative. The only abnormal value was my cholesterol, which was slightly elevated. The doctor said he didn't know what was wrong with me but that my pain was probably related to the way I sit at work."

Barbara continued, "The pain didn't get any better, and I was getting more and more annoyed, so I saw another doctor. Same tests, same results." I looked at the slightly built woman sitting in a stooped position in the chair in my office.

Obviously she was not only in pain but felt very frustrated with the medical profession.

"Barbara, tell me about your lifestyle and your family situation." I pursued this open-ended history-taking, hoping she would reveal things about herself that would help in determining why these symptoms were occurring.

"I grew up in the Midwest," she explained. "My mother was a schoolteacher, and my father was an attorney. I didn't know my father well because he was killed in a plane crash when I was six. My mother remarried, and I didn't like my stepfather at all. He drank a lot and fought with my mother. I realize now that he was abusive. He would walk in on my sister and me when we were dressing or taking a shower. He frequently walked around in just a robe with nothing underneath. I never felt comfortable around him."

"Have you seen a psychologist?" I asked.

"No," she replied sharply, "I'm doing fine without a shrink.

"There was a lot of tension in our home. One of us was always sick with something, and I think the stress had a lot to do with it. My mother always emphasized doing well in school. We were punished if we didn't make good grades. To avoid that, I became very compulsive about studying. I was always serious and didn't spend a lot of time just having fun with my friends. I wanted to be at the top of my class and drove myself to perfection."

"Were you athletic?" I asked.

"No, I really didn't like any sports, and I was in such poor shape physically that, when I tried to run track or play tennis, I just couldn't keep up.

"At any rate," she continued, "I got married after college and then enrolled in law school. I dropped out after the first year because I was so miserable. I put too much pressure on myself.

"Tom and I have two children, and they are wonderful kids. Things began to change though. I began to feel that I couldn't do enough for my family; yet I felt that they took advantage of me, always wanting me to do, but never doing for me."

With her head bowed and her voice cracking, Barbara began to tell me about her symptoms.

"I began to notice that I was tired all the time. I couldn't get enough rest. It was hard to get up in the morning, because even though I slept, it wasn't good restful sleep. Do you know what I mean?" she questioned.

"Yes," I assured her.

"I began to have trouble with cramps and constipation; of course, I wasn't exercising and didn't eat well. My doctor told me that I had irritable bowel syndrome. Have you heard of it?" I acknowledged that I was familiar with irritable bowel problems and was aware that stress is a major contributing factor to its symptoms.

"In the past year, though, my shoulders and back and hips have bothered me the most," she went on. "In the morning, when I get up, it takes me an hour just to stand up straight. I just can't get loose. By the end of the day, I have pain in my neck, shoulders, back, and hips. My son says he feels that way after a football game, but I haven't even gone for a walk. Sometimes my shoulders and hips burn and sting."

"Do you ever stumble or lose your balance?" I asked, trying to see if she had any symptoms of multiple sclerosis.

"No, not really," she replied. "I'm just so worn out, it's the way I felt when I had mononucleosis in high school."

"Did anyone in your family ever have similar complaints?" I asked.

"Now that you mention it," she said after a brief, thoughtful pause, "my mother always complained that her back and hips hurt a lot."

Barbara had no significant gynecologic history. Her periods were normal, and she had no pelvic pain. "Let me examine you to see if I can find anything that is wrong," I said as I pushed the button for my nurse to put the patient in the examination room. When the exam confirmed that there was nothing overtly wrong with Barbara physically, I explained to her what I thought her diagnosis was. "I have seen several women over the past couple of years with findings just like yours, Barbara. I think you may have fibromyalgia. We'll need to have you see a rheumatologist to make sure we're not missing anything else, but I think that this is what is causing your symptoms. Let me tell you about fibromyalgia."

I shared with her some of the following facts.

Fibromyalgia Characteristics

Researchers have found that 15–20 percent of patients seen in a rheumatology clinic actually have fibromyalgia and not rheumatoid arthritis. Eighty percent of these patients are women. It is actually four or five times more common than rheumatoid arthritis.

The disorder is characterized by constant widespread pain so severe it is often incapacitating. Another characteristic is the absence of any definite pathophysiologic change or abnormal laboratory test. The diagnosis is basically made as one of exclusion, that is, all other diagnostic conditions have been ruled out, and only fibromyalgia is left.

This disorder is defined as a condition of muscles, tendons, and attachments to bone that causes stiffness, pain or aching, and localized tender spots. The principal symptoms are chronic fatigue, chronic pain, morning stiffness, and unrefreshing sleep. Sufferers experience a chronic feeling of tiredness and a lack of stamina. The fatigue is worse early in the morning, improves during the day, and gets worse again at night. There is a lack of stamina for repetitive upper extremity exercises. Most patients are not in good physical condition and have never been very athletic.

The pain with fibromyalgia is usually widespread, involving the neck, shoulders, upper back, lower back, and hips. The discomfort is like a deep ache with associated heaviness and sometimes burning. Getting out of bed is a chore, and it often takes several minutes to an hour to loosen up. Once limberness is established, the stiffness abates until later in the day, when a slower pace usually leads to recurrent stiffness.

The symptoms usually occur when the woman is twenty to forty years old, and they are often initiated by an acute sprain, muscle injury, or nerve root irritation (as with a whiplash injury or back strain). Viral illnesses may also predispose a woman to the disorder. Although the pain waxes and wanes, it persists for years. Remission and relapses are very common.

The episodes of intense pain are usually influenced by external factors. For example, cold, rainy weather (it has been theorized that increased barometric pressure increases the thickness of the synovial fluid in the joints, making them stiffer and movement more painful), job stress, marital and family disharmony, and sedentary lifestyle may all precipitate the aches and pains of fibromyalgia. The pain is often severe and debilitating, to the extent that Goldenberg reports that 25.3 percent of women are disabled from work.[1]

Many articles on fibromyalgia describe a characteristic personality type for those with the disease. They are often compulsive, well-organized, extremely serious, self-critical individuals who are perfectionistic, the classic type A personality, women who are often obsessive-compulsive.

Regardless of what the personality type is, fatigue is the principal physical stress that afflicts women with fibromyalgia. This is the tie-in to chronic fatigue syndrome (CFS), which is characterized by intense, long-lasting fatigue and a combination of other symptoms such as muscle weakness, joint pain, and sleep disturbances. As with fibromyalgia, CFS is often initiated with an episode of flulike illness. Symptoms may be very similar to mononucleosis.

Failure to allow sufficient time for sleep is frequent in young, compulsive, perfectionistic people. They often have insomnia, and when they do sleep, it is shallow and not refreshing. Use of caffeine late in the day reduces the body's ability to get uninterrupted, restful sleep. Because they are perfectionistic, they try to press on in spite of the fatigue. They get up tired, it gets worse as the day goes on, and by nighttime, they are exhausted but still can't sleep.

"Does any of this sound familiar, Barbara?" I asked.

"Yes," she replied, "it sounds as if you are telling me my life's story."

The aspect of stress and relaxation brings up a very important point. Time off from duties at work, away from home or in the home, is essential to your well-being. God rested on the seventh day from his creative work and instructed us to do so. A day away from the stresses of the week allows you to relax and decrease the tension and anxiety in your body. When you don't take this time, problems like fibromyalgia can arise.

Women who work at jobs that require repetitive and sustained activity may develop this disorder more easily. Jobs such as typing, using a computer keyboard, working on an assembly line, playing the piano, or doing needlework are the worst. Housework—long hours of cooking, washing, ironing, or vacuuming—make the pain worse. Since most of these patients are not in good physical condition, their muscles are out of shape. Since muscles are unfit and more prone to injury, they are also more prone to simulative trauma and repetitive stress injuries. Therefore changing your situation at work, understanding postural correction, doing flexibility exercises, keeping your spine stable and not bent frequently, and using ice to reduce microtrauma to joints are extremely important.

Until recently, we did not have any specific diagnostic findings for fibromyalgia. Drs. Smythe and Moldofsky now describe "tender points" that patients with fibromyalgia have. They indicate that for a patient to be diagnosed with fibromyalgia, she must have at least eleven of the seventeen points of tenderness present when the areas are palpated on examination. Their research has been supported by several other studies as well.[2]

Points of Tenderness for Fibromyalgia

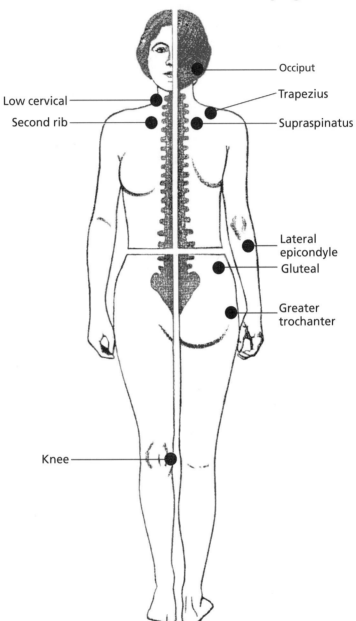

Occiput

Trapezius

Low cervical

Second rib

Supraspinatus

Lateral epicondyle

Gluteal

Greater trochanter

Knee

As you can see in the figure above, tender points are distributed symmetrically on the front and back of the body at points in muscles, tendons, and bony prominences.

Barbara had a look of amazement on her face after we finished our discussion. "It's just such a relief to know that there is a name for the problem I have. I was beginning to think that I was crazy. I hope you haven't told me all of this to tell me there is no cure for fibromyalgia."

"Well, regarding treatment, I have good news and bad news," I replied. "The bad news is that there is no permanent cure. The good news is that if you are willing to work at it, you can see marked improvement in your symptoms, but it will require alteration of your lifestyle. You must begin to see the symptoms as a warning sign that you are fatigued or under too much stress." I continued with an explanation of our current understanding of the management of this disorder.

Managing Fibromyalgia

There is no definitive medical treatment for fibromyalgia or for chronic fatigue syndrome, but several things have been shown to have some benefit in both conditions. It is essential that you become involved in your own treatment by becoming more physically active with regular exercise. Being involved in social activities may help in your effort to reduce stressors.

The key to successful rehabilitation is to return your metabolic system to normal. Those who have written about this disorder emphasize the need for appropriate exercise, diet, and rest.

Since inactivity leads to muscle deconditioning and an increased susceptibility to soreness after exertion, it is important to initiate a regular, medically approved exercise program.

You must begin regular aerobic exercise. I know that as a sufferer of fibromyalgia you don't feel like exercising, and it is not a major interest of yours, but you must start now. You can do aerobics, walking, bicycling, swimming, jogging, power stepping. Whatever you choose, you must do it regularly. Start slowly with five- to ten-minute periods of exercise and build up to three or four times per week for a minimum of thirty minutes. Remember to loosen up five minutes before you begin and cool down five minutes before you finish. If you have any medical illness, be sure to consult your physician before you initiate your program. If you have severe low back pain, neck pain, or upper extremity pain as a part of your symptoms, you may need to be evaluated by an orthopedist or physical therapist to get a regimen of exercises specifically for this area of your body. These would include aerobic conditioning adapted to minimize microtrauma, postural correction, and stretching and flexibility.

You should also have an evaluation made of your work situation and make the necessary adaptations to decrease stress and diminish damaging effects on bones and joints. Work changes may be an essential part of your recovery.

Many women with fibromyalgia or chronic fatigue have poor dietary habits. Eating a well-balanced, nourishing diet is very important. Women should take a multivitamin daily. Some dieticians suggest that additional magnesium is beneficial. Magnesium lactate, in a dose of 84 milligrams a day, would be adequate. If you have heavy menstrual periods, elemental iron in a daily dose of 60–120 milligrams will help to replace iron stores. Calcium, 1,000 milligrams a day between the ages of 40 and 50 and 1,500 milligrams a day after age 50, should be taken to help keep your bones strong.

Adequate, restful sleep is very important as an aid to improvement in symptoms. This is especially important when you sense that the symptoms are getting worse. The antidepressant medication amitriptyline (Elavil) is often beneficial in affecting mood and allowing for adequate restful sleep.

There are other important things for you to do. You must begin to identify the stresses in your life and deal with them in a manner that allows you to modify or eliminate them. Get the sleep that you need, but remember, excessive sleep is not beneficial.

You may have tried different pain pills and found that they are not very effective. This is not uncommon at all. In spite of this, reports indicate that 97 percent of fibromyalgia patients take pain medication. Of all the medications tried, nonsteroidal, anti-inflammatory agents such as ibuprofen are probably the best. Remember that these medications can irritate your stomach.

Some patients indicate a positive response to transcutaneous electrical nerve stimulation (TENS) units. TENS works by blocking the pain, which in turn allows you to stop guarding and having muscle spasms. When you stop having spasms, you experience a real reduction in pain and have an opportunity for microtrauma healing.

Other patients may require steroid injections at some of the most tender points.

Although sleeping medication and strong narcotic pain medicines do not consistently result in improvement of the pain, antidepressants may be beneficial in improving sleep patterns and relieving some of the severe pain. Getting into a counseling situation with a trained psychologist or psychiatrist who understands the interaction of stress and fibromyalgia can be very beneficial.

If you are like most patients, you will have periods of improvement and periods of relapse with the pain. Usually, something has changed. You stopped exercising, had a severe bout with the flu, or had a stressful event in your life or that of someone close to you. Don't panic; get in touch with yourself and determine what has changed to cause your recurrence. Go back to the basics of treatment and you will find that your pain will decrease again, although you may never be totally pain free.

I prayed with Barbara that she would find the spiritual resources from God to resolve the stress in her life and that her pain would decrease. Then I gave her a list developed by Dr. Paul Davidson, from San Francisco, that outlines the treatment of fibromyalgia. He uses the acronym RETRAIN.[3]

Rest and relaxation
Educate yourself about your condition
Therapeutic muscle training
Revamping your response to stress
Analgesics and
Injections at very tender points
Never give up hope

As Barbara left, I noticed that she wasn't quite as stooped, and she had a smile on her face. The thank-you note I received three months later, indicating her significant improvement, gave me a great feeling of satisfaction. Treatment doesn't have to come from a bottle of pills or a surgical scalpel.

Let not your heart be troubled; believe in God, believe also in Me.

John 14:1

A Spiritual Perspective

I have fibromyalgia. I know the frustration of inexplicable pain, the nebulous symptoms that make you sound more like a hypochondriac than a person who is genuinely suffering. As David has said, only in recent years have physicians in fields outside of rheumatology begun to respect the whole package of symptoms called fibromyalgia as a legitimate diagnosis.

For a long time I was embarrassed to tell anyone how genuinely bad I felt all the time. I had been chronically fatigued for so long it was starting to seem normal. The ice-pick pain in every quadrant of my body disturbed my sleep and made me feel cranky and very old. I was afraid that I actually had multiple sclerosis or lupus. I felt afraid to see a doctor and afraid not to. My own doctor-husband knew relatively little about fibromyalgia until I was finally diagnosed by a rheumatologist and a physical therapist about five years ago.

I am a Christian who believes deeply in the healing power of the Holy Spirit, but I have not been able to pray away my fibromyalgia. What I have been able to do is go to the Lord and ask him to teach me the meaning of healthy self-care. Like most mothers, I instinctively know how to nurture others, but I am often poor at loving myself. Yet, doesn't the Word tell us to "love your neighbor as yourself"? As early as in Leviticus 19:18 we find this teaching. Go to Galatians and find that Paul says "the entire law is summed up in this single command"! Matthew, Mark, Luke, Romans, and James all repeat this command in virtually identical wording. My Bible professors tell me that when God goes to the trouble of mentioning something more than once in his Word, we should heed the teaching as one that is vital to our well-being.

Leviticus 25:18–21 (NIV) says: "Follow my decrees and be careful to obey my laws, and you will live safely in the land. Then the land will yield its fruit, and you will eat your fill and live there in safety. . . . I will send you . . . a blessing." Please observe that the children of God did not have to go to another land to receive his help, instruction, and blessing; he blessed them right where they were living. And so it is with those of us who are living with fibromyalgia (and any other physical problems). I do not rule out the possibility of and certainly not the power of God in healing any of us, supernaturally, at any moment of his choosing. However, if that has not yet been your experience, let me encourage you to look for his hand of mercy in the midst of your present circumstances.

Isaiah 41:10 tells us not to fear or to be dismayed, because our God is going to strengthen us and help us and uphold us with his righteous right hand. God doesn't love any one of us more than he loves every one of us. Stay in Isaiah and turn to chapter 48, verses 17–18(NIV): "I am the LORD your God, who teaches you what is best for you, who directs you in the way you should go. If only you had paid attention to my commands, your peace would have been like a river." My friend, in all the years I have walked with the Lord, and they number more than forty, I have never seen him fail to give me wisdom when I am willing to pay the price in obedience. If you are stuck and can't seem to get through a tough place, go back to your last place of disobedience, and you will find the Lord waiting there for you. When you have completed that task of obedience, he will give you more instruction.

After reading David's chapter on fibromyalgia, you know that it is primarily a stress-related disorder. I do not know what particular things the Lord will ask you to do to lower your stress level, but I know that he will instruct if you take the time to listen and are willing to be obedient, even in the things that may seem insignificant to you. A life marked by abundance and victory is built from the small bricks of obedience to the seemingly insignificant. As we obey the Lord, he constructs for us a sure foundation, built on the solid rock of his Word and wisdom, and we move into healing and wholeness as a process. It's the journey, not the destination, that should be our focus. I am moving in less pain, experiencing deeper rest, and learning to just say no to many, many opportunities and worthy endeavors, as the Lord instructs me. It's a daily experience. There is fresh mercy for each new day. No stale manna for God's people!

Scriptures for Meditation

Leviticus 19:18
Matthew 19:19
Mark 12:31
Luke 10:27
Romans 13:9
Galatians 5:14
James 2:8

From the pages of the Old Testament to the end of the New Testament the message is repeated. Over and over again God is trying to make something very clear to us. What is the message? We can never love others as they need to be loved until we have first learned how to love ourselves. Exactly what is involved in loving yourself?

Can you be a servant of the Lord and love yourself at the same time?

Suggested Spiritual Exercise

Make a list of every activity in which you are involved or for which you bear some responsibility. For wives and mothers, this should include those related to your children and your husband's career. If you are single, include things you do for people in your office, your parents, friends, boyfriend, girlfriends, pets—whoever. The idea here is for you to get a full picture of all that you have loaded onto your plate in the buffet line of life. Now, take this list with you to your chosen place of prayer. If you want to make a real ceremony out of this, write each activity or responsibility on a separate strip of paper and put them all in a basket. Light a candle or sit in front of a warm fire and ask the Lord which of these pieces of paper should stay in your basket and which of them should go into the fire. Meditate on the answers you feel you receive for several days and then methodically begin eliminating those activities that are taking you over the edge.

Don't expect to get any thank-you notes from the people you may need to disappoint. Make a mental note about how you feel doing this and respect (and maybe even compliment) others when they must say no to you. This is between you and the Lord, and it really doesn't matter how many others truly understand. I just tell people the dead-level truth: "I'm going under, and I must cut back."

Most people will envy your courage, and surely the Lord will begin to bless you in ways you can't even imagine just now.

8

TMJ Disorder

Many of the stress-related disorders that I describe in this book are great mimickers. In other words, their symptoms resemble the symptoms of other diseases. Fibromyalgia causes symptoms similar to arthritis; irritable bowel syndrome has symptoms similar to inflammatory bowel disease. Another such disorder is temporomandibular joint (TMJ) disorder, which frequently presents with symptoms very similar to an earache or a migraine headache.

I recall hearing about TMJ disorder in medical school, but it certainly didn't seem like a serious disorder. I really didn't become aware of what a significant problem this is until I heard a noted otolaryngologist—ear, nose, and throat specialist—discuss the frequency of TMJ problems and how often they are misdiagnosed. Since then I have considered this as a diagnosis whenever women are seen in the office with complaints of persistent or recurrent earache, sinus problems with pain in the area of the ear, or persistent headaches on the side of the head above the ear. I have referred many patients with TMJ dysfunction to ear, nose, and throat specialists. One such patient is Phyllis Kane.

Phyllis is a thirty-one-year-old woman who recently came to me as a new patient. She was referred because her family physician had obtained a Pap smear that indicated that she had dysplasia of the cervix with associated changes indicating human papilloma virus (HPV) infection.

Dysplasia is considered to be a premalignant change in the cells of the cervix. Pap smears can be read as normal, atypical (meaning the cells are not completely normal but are not yet bad enough to be abnormal), or dysplastic (meaning the surface cells are definitely abnormal). Dysplasia can be classified as mild, moderate, or severe. The abnormality then progresses to localized cancer cells, called carcinoma insitu (CIS), and then to frankly invasive cancer.

Human papilloma virus is a sexually transmitted viral organism that frequently infects the genitalia of men and women. Each year there are estimated to be over four million cases of HPV in the United States. Some strains of the virus cause large genital warts, which may occur on the penis, scrotum, and groin in men, as well as in the urethra or rectum. In women, warts may appear on the vulva, groin, perineum, and anus as well as in the vagina, urethra, and rectum. Other strains may cause what are called flat warts, which infect the vulva, vagina, and cervix. These areas of infection may subsequently develop abnormal or dysplastic cells. HPV is associated with over 90 percent of all cervical dysplasia and cancer in women.

Phyllis is a sales manager who had been married to a child psychologist. They have a son who is now nine years old. In the course of obtaining medical history from Phyllis, she indicated that she felt she had been infected by her former husband.

"I really thought we had a great marriage," Phyllis said to me. "We spent time together; we frequently traveled together to his meetings and had great family vacations. Mike was an ideal husband. He was so thoughtful and kind; he pampered me in a way that most women want to be spoiled. But one day, he came home from work and said he didn't love me anymore and that he wanted a divorce.

"I was flabbergasted," Phyllis went on. "I had no idea that he was unhappy. I know that sounds very naive, but it's true. I still don't know why he left. I think he hit midlife and had to prove his virility and attractiveness again.

"About six months after he left, I began to notice these bumps on my vulva. They caused some itching but really didn't hurt much at all. I was treated with a topical solution on the warts, and they resolved. One year later, I had a Pap smear by my family doctor, and it indicated that I had dysplasia of the cervix. He told me that I had probably acquired the virus from my former husband. I felt like killing Mike, then.

"He had the nerve to pretend everything was okay, while he was having an affair, and he left without any explanation. He infected me with his girlfriend's virus, and now I may have dysplasia. I don't deserve this. He's not suffering at all, and I'll suffer the consequences for life."

Phyllis had a microscopic procedure done, called colposcopy, which revealed abnormal cells of the cervix. Biopsies confirmed severe dysplasia. She then had a carbon-dioxide laser procedure to destroy the affected cervical tissue.

As I was evaluating and treating Phyllis's cervical HPV problem, she began to express other complaints. Frequent, nagging headaches located above her right ear were more and more of a problem. She also complained of recurrent earaches and ringing in her ear, again on the right side. The stress of her divorce, cervical dysplasia, and recurrent pain in the right ear and side of the head was definitely taking a toll on this young single parent.

Phyllis had been treated for infection in the ear on three occasions, with no improvement in her symptoms. She was also taking a medication for supposed migraine headaches and saw no improvement with that either.

I might not have figured out Phyllis's problem had she not been in my office late one afternoon for a Pap smear to make sure her cervical dysplasia was effectively treated. She had been busy at her office and obviously felt tired. As I stood beside the exam table, jotting notes onto her chart, she yawned. I was startled by the loud pop I heard as she opened her mouth. It was almost like the sound of a branch breaking. Her jaw cracked loudly, but Phyllis didn't even seem to notice. Suddenly, it dawned on me what the source of her pain and headaches was.

"Phyllis," I asked, "does your jaw always pop like that?"

"Oh, yes," she replied, "but it's nothing, it really doesn't hurt that much."

"Do you ever find yourself grinding your teeth?" I asked.

"No," she said, "but my ex-husband used to say that I did grind my teeth in my sleep all the time."

"Phyllis, I think I know what your problem is."

"You think I'm mentally ill," she replied in jest.

"No," I emphasized, "I think you may have TMJ disorder. You know, temporomandibular joint disorder."

"No, I don't know," she said, "tell me about it." I began to tell her about TMJ disorder and its associated symptoms and signs.

How the TMJ Works

Though you seldom think about your temporomandibular joint (TMJ), it is one of the most frequently used areas of your body. Every time you chew or talk or swallow (one of which occurs approximately once in every three minutes), you use your TMJ.

Located at the point where the lower jaw—the mandible—joins the skull at the temporal bone, the TMJ is immediately in front of the ear on either side of the head. You can locate the joint by putting your finger on the triangular structure in front of your ear, moving your finger slightly forward, and pressing firmly while you open your jaw all the way and then shut it. This movement or motion that you feel is the joint. If you have temporomandibular dysfunction, you will experience discomfort when you do this maneuver.

The TMJ acts as a lever (the jaw) and fulcrum (the joint). When you bite down forcefully, you not only put force on the object between your teeth, but also on the joint. Studies have shown that there is more force applied per square inch to the surface of the joint than to whatever is between your teeth. Fortunately, God designed this joint to be able to accommodate the daily wear and tear that it undergoes by making it a sliding joint rather than the common ball-and-socket type. This joint, like others, is lined with a rubbery, slippery material called cartilage, which allows for smooth motion and function. As such, the forces generated by chewing, talking, and swallowing can be distributed over a wider surface in the joint space. This dissipates the wear and tear and allows time for repair to occur rapidly, especially between chewing.

Groups of muscles that contract and relax so that you can open and close your mouth to talk and chew affect your TMJ. It is also affected by your bite or the way your upper and lower teeth align and also by the bones in your jaw. In order to function appropriately and effectively, the muscles must be able to relax and work in a balanced manner. Your teeth must be well aligned and your bite stable with teeth coming together properly. The joints themselves must open and close comfortably and be free of degenerating disease or injury. In other words, all of these things must work in synchrony.

Stress and TMJ Disorder

So what happens if you don't have synchrony? Stress, grinding or clenching of the teeth, and faulty posture can cause your muscles to tighten up and put undue pressure on the TMJ. Malocclusion, when the teeth come together poorly, also places repetitive stress on the joint. Injury to the joint itself, such as occurs in accidents or with a degenerating disease like arthritis, can result in abnormal function.

How does stress fit into this picture of TMJ dysfunction? Stressed persons have a tendency to do things repetitively that result in loss of synchrony of this strategic joint. Under stress, muscles tighten, jaws clench, teeth are ground, meals are eaten rapidly, gum is chewed, and excessive pressure is placed on the TMJ without an adequate amount of time in between to allow repair of the cartilage to occur.

First, you must identify actions that may be causing dysfunction. Many people who grind or grit their teeth are unaware of it unless someone tells them, just as in Phyllis's case. If you always chew your food on one side, you may put excessive pressure on one joint, instead of equally dividing the pressure, as you do when you alternate sides when you chew.

Obviously, all TMJ dysfunction is not stress related. Malocclusion of the teeth, resulting in an improper bite, is a developmental problem and not a result of stress. Injury to the joint or degenerative changes from disease cannot necessarily be changed by decreasing stress (although the problem may cause more stress).

TMJ Disorder Symptoms

How do you feel when you have TMJ problems? The pain of TMJ dysfunction is quite variable. For some it is sharp and searing, for others it is more dull and achy. The pain is usually focused over the joint, immediately in front of the ear. It may radiate out from this site. Some people have constant pain, although for most it is noted when they chew, talk, swallow, or yawn.

The pain often causes spasm in the adjacent muscles attached to the bones of the skull, face, and jaws. Thus, the pain can be felt along the side of the head in front of and above the ear, the cheek, the lower jaw, and the teeth.

The most frequently perceived location of pain is in the ear. Because of this, many patients present for care with complaints of an ear infection. On examination, however, the eardrum is normal, with no fluid behind it. There is also no alteration of hearing. The popping or clicking noise that occurs when the jaw is opened clinches the diagnosis. Some individuals cannot open their jaws completely due to the pain that results from the chronic irritation in the joint.

Management of TMJ Dysfunction

Reducing Joint Injury	Encouraging Joint Healing
Keep teeth apart	Ice joint acutely
Avoid grinding or clenching teeth	Apply heat to joint
Avoid chewing gum or hard candy	Use buffered aspirin or anti-inflammatory agents
Chew evenly on both sides of mouth	Exercise joint
Avoid hard, chewy foods	Use braces or orthopedic appliances
Practice good posture	
Reduce stress	
Use anti-inflammatory agents	

The treatment of TMJ dysfunction is intended to relieve your pain and centers on stress management and reducing the amount of wear and tear on the joint. You can rest the TMJ by keeping your teeth apart to avoid grinding your teeth; chewing evenly on both sides of the mouth; avoiding chewing gum, hard candy, or hard, chewy foods; and practicing good posture. Keeping your teeth apart relaxes your jaw and prevents grinding of the teeth. Good posture of the head, neck, and back assists in keeping the jaw properly positioned. Eating soft foods helps to decrease wear and tear on the joint.

Promote healing through the use of ice alternating with heat, taking anti-inflammatory agents, and exercising. At the time of an acute flare-up of pain in the TMJ, ice should be applied to decrease swelling. Thereafter, heat (in the form of moist, hot towels or a moist heating pad) should be used to relax tense muscles. Anti-inflammatory medications such as aspirin or ibuprofen-type agents can decrease pain and inflammation. Exercises restore flexibility to the joint. Opening and closing the mouth while keeping your teeth aligned helps to strengthen involved muscles. Exercises should only be done for a few minutes once or twice a day.

Since stress is so frequently a predisposing factor in TMJ dysfunction, it is imperative that steps be taken to reduce the stressors in your life. Many patients are totally unaware that stress is a factor in the pain they experience in the jaw. Relaxation techniques, use of biofeedback (the technique of making bodily processes, such as heartbeats, perceptible to the senses in order to consciously control them) to help you control your body's responses to stress, and counseling may all be beneficial.

If your pain is not relieved by any of the above techniques, see your dentist or orthodontist. Several types of devices can be designed to help restore normal anatomy and re-

lieve pain. Guards or retainers can be worn at night to prevent grinding or clenching of the teeth. Repositioning appliances are used to realign the jaw and must be worn
twenty-four hours a day. When necessary, placement of a
bridge or crown may stabilize your bite. Use of braces, as
well as retainers, may be necessary to restore proper align-
ment of teeth and the TMJ. Sometimes an otolaryngologist
or oral-facial surgeon will be needed to repair your joint.
Often this can be done by use of an instrument called an
arthroscope, avoiding large incisions on the face and neck.

Phyllis was treated by instituting relaxation techniques,
counseling, and ibuprofen. Her symptoms improved but
were not completely relieved. An orthodontist fitted her
with a retainer, ending her ability to grind her teeth at
night, and her symptoms abated.

Remember that stress is a major contributing factor in
TMJ dysfunction. Stress can affect every body system, and
frequently multiple systems are involved.

A Spiritual Perspective

In Luke 19:37–40, we come upon Jesus walking along
the road; people are spreading out their cloaks to wel-
come him. The whole crowd of disciples is praising God
for all of the miracles they have seen him do through Jesus.
The Pharisees tell Jesus to rebuke his disciples, since they
believe the disciples' praise is blasphemous. Instead Jesus
rebukes the Pharisees by saying, "I tell you if these become silent, the stones will cry out!"

There is a miracle at work even in the dysfunction of our
bodies. God, our Creator, has built into our bodies something that is also inherent to nature. His creation is meant to
testify to his kingship over every living thing and to his hand

at work in every detail of living. We are not meant to live wrong and have it turn out right. If we do not understand this, our loving God, in his prevenient grace, will go ahead of us and behind us causing everything, even the rocks, to vie for our attention. When our bodies begin to ache, we do well to get the message as early as possible. Early detection can lead to cure of more than just cancer. The sooner we heed the message hidden in our pain, the sooner we can begin to move into the healing the Holy Spirit has for us.

Scripture for Meditation

Luke 19:41–44

Read the meditation verses and think of yourself as "Jerusalem." When you are sick and in pain, the Spirit of God is weeping over you. He is acquainted with your pain, and he would say to you, even as he said to Jerusalem so long ago: "If only you knew what would bring you peace." Jesus is teaching us in this passage that if we do not recognize his lordship over our lives, we and the generations after us will be adversely affected—and all for one seemingly simple error on our parts: we do not recognize the time of God coming to us.

A Suggested Prayer

Lord Jesus, help me to see you through the veil of pain that blinds my eyes. What is the message hidden in my suffering? I recognize that you, O Lord, are the only One who fully knows what will bring me peace. Let the pain and sickness of dysfunction end with me and my generation. Give me discerning eyes and ears so that I may hear, and hearing, obey and obeying, live in wholeness and newness of life through Christ, our Lord. Amen.

9

The Immune System

This is the most difficult chapter in this book to write—not because it required research, although I made an extensive review of the current literature to gather this information. Much of our current understanding of the interaction between stress and the immune system has come from research done in the past decade, and the field continues to expand. It was difficult because I have tried to be sensitive to your feelings. I know that you or someone you love may have cancer or some immune disorder. When you read that stress may play a role in precipitating abnormal function of the immune system, making it difficult to combat an illness such as cancer, you may become very upset. You realize that the persons you love very much who have cancer might have been able to help themselves by dealing with life's stresses in a more functional manner. My mother and my mother-in-law, both of whom had cancer, found it upsetting that stress may have played a role in their susceptibility to malignant disease.

Not all physicians, psychiatrists, and psychologists will agree with this information. However, there is more and more information in the literature to support these concepts. Studies by renowned immunology researchers point to a definite link between stress and immune suppression. A paper by Khansari reported, "Stress, distress and a variety of psychiatric illnesses, notably the affective disorders, are increasingly reported to be associated with immunosuppression."

We cannot change the effects that stress had on those who have cancer, but perhaps your understanding of what stress does to your immune system will help you avoid some of its detrimental consequences.

I want to make it very clear that I am not saying that stress causes cancer. I am saying that the manner in which one deals with stress may influence the ability to combat carcinogenic effects.

Perhaps Janice's story will help you understand this association. We cannot prove that personality type and stress contributed to Janice's cancer, but current research certainly indicates it is possible.

Janice had been a patient in my practice for ten years. I saw her for routine exams, including Pap smears and mammograms, and also for frequent recurrences of vaginal infection, upper respiratory infections such as colds and flu, and persistent flare-ups of irritable bowel syndrome. I got to know her well, and over time, she revealed interesting aspects of her personal history to me.

"My family was very religious when I was growing up, almost puritanical in their approach. We were always in church, whether we wanted to be or not. I recognize now the benefits of a Christian home, but I also see the detrimental effects of being so legalistic. I was taught to be quiet unless spoken to, to keep my feelings to myself, not to express anger, and to always do what I was told without questioning it. There is also another piece of information that I couldn't even talk about until recently—I was sexually abused by a man who was a family friend and who lived in our home when I was a child. As a result of all of this, I turned in on myself, because that was the only safe place for me.

"As I moved into my high school and college years, my personality was significantly affected by all of this childhood trauma. I never did anything bad, because I was afraid to. I was always doing things to make other people feel good, and then I was angry because I felt used, but I couldn't express my anger. I was always nice, but I didn't feel nice; I felt dirty and ugly and undesirable."

This was the background that Janice relayed to me during her office visits. She was anxious and high strung, had frequent panic attacks, and seemed to be ill all the time. I became suspicious that Janice had a major problem when she came for an annual checkup. She looked tired and drawn, her color wasn't good, and she complained that she was noticing blood in her urine. I examined her and did a Pap smear, which was negative for malignant cells. A recent mammogram was also negative.

Because of the bleeding, I referred Janice to a urologist. He performed cystoscopy (looking into the bladder with a lighted instrument), and diagnosed a large bladder cancer. Radical surgery followed to remove the tumor, and it was felt that she would have a good result.

In spite of chemotherapy, however, Janice was dead thirteen months later.

Is Janice's story unusual? No, unfortunately there are many young women with cancer. Bladder cancer is not as common as breast, lung, cervical, uterine, ovarian, and colon cancer. The connection, however, between marked stress and the way it is handled is a topic of current interest among researchers. Let me give you some of the most recent information.

Immunity Update

The body's immune system is the lymphatic system. It is comprised primarily of the lymph nodes, tonsils, thymus, spleen, and lymphatic vessels. It is designed to protect the integrity of the body from outside invasion. When confronted with infectious organisms or anything perceived to be foreign, it manifests what is called an immune response, by producing *antibodies* to fight the foreign invader.

This system of recognition is called *self* and *nonself.* The body of a normal healthy woman does not recognize any of her own cells as foreign and does not produce antibodies to these cells. This is self. Anything that is not a part of her body system would be considered nonself, and her body would produce antibodies to attack and destroy the foreign material or organisms. When the immune system produces antibodies to destroy its own cells, this is called an auto-immune disorder. Examples of such diseases are rheumatoid arthritis and lupus.

An effective immune system depends on a highly mobile population of cells in the lymphatic system. The lymphatic system is, in essence, the river of immune factors that flows through the body in a system of interconnecting vessels called lymphatics.

Lymphocytes, a class of white blood cells, produce antibodies. Certain diseases can affect these cells and alter their balance. AIDS, for example, is caused by a retrovirus, HIV-I, that attacks lymphocytes, thereby damaging the body's ability to fight disease.

Recent research indicates a close connection between adaptive responses involving the central nervous system and immune outcome. Jankovic has described phenomena that support the contention that there are numerous and continuous intercommunications between the nervous system and the immune system.

If these data are true, then anything that affects the central nervous system can have an impact on the body's ability to fight disease—nonself. Depression, for example, can affect normal central nervous system hormonal production and thus have an impact on the immune system. Protein malnutrition affects all body systems, including the central nervous system. Malnutrition is considered to be one of the most frequent causes of failure of the immune system in the world today.

Chapter 1 described the release of steroids from the adrenal glands in response to stress. These steroids can directly alter the normal immune response in the body. Stress can affect the body chemicals that control the migration of lymph cells so they cannot reach their target as effectively. Ottaway has also shown that stress can alter the normal migration patterns of lymphocytes and diminish the effectiveness of the immune system. Stress then not only contributes to the development of various diseases in the body, but also inhibits the ability of the body to fight disease. This is more evidence to indicate that stress makes us sick.

Stress Effects on the Immune System

Affects central nervous system control of migration of lymphocytes

Affects central nervous system hormonal production, altering immune system

Alters steroid release from adrenal glands, altering immune response

Affects self, nonself recognition

Lowers ability of cells to resist invasion

Diminishes effectiveness of immune system

Behavioral oncologists, reports Baltrusch, have conceptualized a type C cancer risk pattern. Much as a type A personality predisposes a person to an increased risk of cardiovascular disease, the type C personality predisposes a patient to an increased risk of malignant disease.

This personality pattern features denial and suppression of emotions—particularly anger. It involves pathological niceness, avoidance of conflicts, exaggerated social desirability, harmonizing behavior, overcompliance, high rationality, and a rigid control of emotional expression. This pattern is usually concealed behind a pattern of pleasantness and appears to be effective as long as a relatively stable environmental and psychological state is maintained.

This pattern of defense collapses under the impact of accumulated strains and stresses. We find this especially true for those stresses that evoke depression, helplessness, and hopelessness.

Prominent coping features mentioned by Baltrusch include excessive denial, avoidance, and suppression and repression of emotions and basic needs. These coping mechanisms appear to weaken the individual's resistance to carcinogenic influences. They may be linked to the development of tumors and alterations of the body's defense mechanisms against cancer. Stresses that alter the body's normal ability to combat disease may predispose stressed women to a greater risk of developing malignancies.

In another recent study, Born reported that attacking cells (cells that may cause disease) may be able to distinguish between stressed and nonstressed cells. This means that on a level as small as the cell, precursors of malignancy may actually choose the cells they will attack, based on how stressed and damaged they are.

When we combine the facts that one in ten Americans suffer from anxiety-related disorders and that stress is one of the leading causes for visits to doctors' offices today, considering the exposure in our environment to numerous cancer-causing agents, is there any wonder that we see so many women with cancer?

In addition to environmental stresses, there is also the additional anxiety of knowing that there is a family history of cancer. The triad of breast, colon, and ovarian cancer are often seen in a familial distribution. These cancers are known as *adenocarcinomas,* or glandular-type tumors. It is not unusual to see these three types of cancer distributed among the women when a family tree is sketched out.

A strong family history would include a mother or sisters with cancer of the breast, colon, or ovary. Even then, if your mother developed cancer of the breast after the age of menopause, your risk is less than if she was diagnosed before menopause.

There is extensive research being done to evaluate the genetics of cancer. More and more evidence indicates that there are genetic factors that cause suppression of the growth of malignant cells or that prevent suppression. Factors such as diet, environmental carcinogens, infections, and so forth may accentuate these genetic conditions.

What can you do to alter these events? Obviously you can do nothing about the family into which you were born, but if there is a strong family history of cancer, be sure that you have regular examinations. The current American College of Radiology recommendations are for a baseline mammogram between ages thirty-five and forty, regular mammograms every two years from forty to fifty, then yearly thereafter. If your mother or a sister was diagnosed with breast cancer at an age less than thirty-five years old, you should begin your mammograms even earlier. If your family history is positive for colon cancer, you should have colonoscopy (looking into the colon with a lighted scope) at age forty, and thereafter as recommended by your physician. No good screening test for ovarian cancer currently exists. The use of ultrasound scans to screen the ovaries is now being evaluated in research studies, to determine if it is a cost-effective measure for detecting ovarian cancer at earlier stages. There are no reliable blood tests to diagnose any of these cancers.

Cancers of the breast, colon, and ovary are all very difficult to diagnose in an early stage of disease. Of these, ovarian cancer is more frequently not detected until an advanced stage. It is extremely important to be diligent about monthly breast self-exams, reporting any changes or unusual lumps to your physician. You should have regular pelvic exams and Pap smears and report any unusual mucus or blood from the rectum. A well-balanced diet, regular exercise, and avoidance of excessive stress are also very important. Taking time to meditate and pray, to reflect quietly, and to learn to live in faith and obedience to God will help you minimize your stress.

> Let heaven fill your thoughts; don't spend your time worrying about things down here.
>
> Colossians 3:2 TLB

A Spiritual Perspective

My mother fought her final battle with breast cancer in the last eight months of 1994, crossing over into her heavenly assignment on December 29, 1994. Her immune system was no longer able to protect the integrity of her body from the outside invasion of cancer cells.

When the arm of flesh failed her, the right hand of God upheld her in miraculous ways. Some of you who are reading this book have cancer, and you need the comfort of this testimony.

David and I were Mother's primary caregivers during these final eight months of her life, and we saw God give her peaceful sleep, release from pain, and freedom from fear. She experienced the literal presence of angels. In the end, she left this earth just as she prayed she would: she died very peacefully in her sleep, surrounded by people who loved her, and without pain or distress. God does not love anyone more than he loves everyone, and what he did for my mother, he will also do for you.

Mother was diagnosed with breast cancer in 1977. Prayerfully, she followed her oncologist's advice and took advantage of all the surgery, chemotherapy, and radiation that were available. To human wisdom, God added his own touch, and she had seventeen very good years. She liked to say, "I'm not dying of cancer; I am living with cancer."

Despite all we do to lower stress and live in obedience to God, we too may find ourselves the victims of life-threatening diseases. We live in a fallen, sinful world, and disease is a part of that package. We live in this evil world, but we Christians do not live as ones without hope. Our temporary living conditions on this planet have to be seen with an eye to the eternal. Life itself is a terminal condition.

If the Lord Jesus came today, would he claim you as one of his own?

Scriptures for Meditation

1 Thessalonians 4:13
Ephesians 1:18–23

Titus 1:1–2; 2:13–15; 3:7
Hebrews 3
1 Peter 1

Once again the Word of God repeats a message over and over again. We know then that the Spirit of God is seeking to implant a very important, even life-changing, truth in our hearts and minds. Our heavenly Father knows we all dread and fear the grave but he wants us to be born again into the *living hope of resurrection.* We Christians are not to live as people who have no hope; all our hope is found in him.

Since I have so recently had the privilege of walking up to the edge of the other side with my mother and with my mother-in-law I have seen something of the dying grace that the blessed Holy Spirit gives to his own.

We see death as the ultimate curse, but in actuality it is the ultimate blessing since it takes those who know Christ into a realm where we are freed from the bondage to the limited capabilities of our human frames. We are released into a love that is unspeakable! Death in Christ is the great enabler. At last we are able to love as we have been loved and to know as we have been known. Those who are left behind grieve, and rightly so, but we Christians need never be captive to a crippling fear of our own death experience. That kind of fear comes from the pit of hell, and we need to rebuke Satan when he tries to lay it on us. I now know that when the moment of my own death comes I will be given all the grace I need and more. No sting! No victorious grave!

Let these Scripture passages build an eternal hope in your heart. You *will not be disappointed.*

A Suggested Prayer

Lord Jesus, even the thought of finding cancer in my body fills me with a fear that only you can conquer. It is so good to know that you have not given me a spirit of fear but of power and of a sound mind (see 2 Tim. 1:7 KJV). Help me to look to you, my blessed Savior, for the strength and courage I need to live this day. I know that your mercies are new every morning and that your strength is sufficient for every need I have had, have now, or ever will have. By your grace, I determine this day to put away self-condemnation, unwarranted guilt, and all fear. As an act of my will, I choose to trust an unknown future to the God of the universe. Believing you will never leave me or forsake me in any circumstance, I surrender myself and all those whom I love so dearly into your loving care.

10

Eating Disorders

*I*f you are significantly underweight or overweight, you are going to be tempted to turn to the next chapter. All you need is another lecture on how to gain weight or how to lose weight, right? Well, hold on, this is not a critical, shaming discussion about under- or overeating. This chapter is intended to help you understand what eating disorders are and how frequently they occur. Stress plays an important role in initiating and perpetuating eating disorders. I will make suggestions for appropriate nutrition and exercise. So don't leaf ahead. This information may help you recognize and resolve a problem that you haven't been able to resolve before.

Weight Problems

Reports indicate that thirty-four million Americans are overweight. A smaller, but equally impressive number are underweight, based on ideal body-weight or body-mass-index scales. Life insurance actuarial tables for height and weight may be very misleading. They indicate the weight at which one would be expected to live the longest, but they are calculated for groups, not individuals. Actually, persons who are slightly overweight live the longest of any group.

Society defines ideal weights for us by glorifying model-like dimensions, rarely publicizing the manipulations those individuals frequently go through to maintain this ideal weight.

Recent research indicates that we each have a set point weight that is unique. This set point is the weight that the body prefers and will attempt to maintain. Set points are a result of genetic influences and diet and lifestyles. At times they may be overridden and changed. For example, obese persons have set points that are higher than recognized ideal body weights, and it is beneficial for these set points to be returned to normal.

Measures of normal weight are quite variable. Height/weight tables are used by insurance companies and are based on longevity data. "The Twenties Test" says that your ideal weight is attained in your twenties and you should not get more than 10 percent above that weight. If you get more than 20 percent above that weight, you are obese. "The Pinch Test" says you are overweight if you can pinch one inch of flesh in your waist when you are upright.

Ideal body weight used in tables is for average weights at given ages. You are overweight or underweight if you are 10–19 percent from ideal, and obese or pathologically thin if you are more than 20 percent from ideal. The body mass index is defined by your weight (in kilograms) divided by your height (in meters) squared ($\frac{W}{H^2} = BMI$). Normal is 20–26. Obesity is 29 or greater, excessive thinness is 15 or less.

All of these scales are difficult to understand. A very simple way to calculate your ideal body weight is the 5-pounds-per-inch formula. Allow 100 pounds for 5 feet in height, then allow 5 pounds for every inch above 5 feet (i.e., the ideal body weight for a 5'5" woman would be 125 pounds). For large-framed women, allow a 10 percent excess and for a small frame, subtract 10 percent.

Regardless of what ideal weight might be, the fact is contemporary Western society accepts only one standard as ideal—thinness. "Be thin and fit and smile happily while trying to get there." "Be thin, athletic, and active, and you will be considered beautiful." We hear about eating well, but if the major emphasis is on getting thin, you will eat less frequently and often in an unhealthy way.

There is some recent evidence that some individuals who are obese have a genetic predisposition toward excessive weight. If this is true, then detecting those persons and intervening with dietary counseling and exercise advice early in life may be beneficial.

Women tend not to worry so much about the consequences of persistent weight gain or loss, but concentrate on the acute effects on their appearance. There are, however, serious disease states that occur in the lives of individuals who are excessively under- or overweight.

Obesity approximately triples the risks of developing diabetes, hypertension (elevated blood pressure), hyperlipidemia (elevated triglycerides and cholesterol), and cardiovascular disease. If the distribution of fat is upper body or abdominal, the risks of these disease states are greater than if the area of excessive weight is in the lower body.

The effects of excessive thinness include menstrual disorders, anxiety-related disorders, and altered immunity.

You may be saying, "But I don't have a weight problem, and I never will." If not, you are very fortunate. The majority of men and women have more and more difficulty controlling their weight as they get older. Brown studied 41,184 women over time and found that the average weight gain between 18 and 50 years of age is 24.3 pounds. Many women blame this weight gain on pregnancy, but this same study showed that the average additional weight maintained after each pregnancy was only 1.2 pounds.[1] The usual contributing factors are the absence of regular, vigorous exercise, failure to control dietary intake, and stress. So most of us struggle with weight as we age. Women also have to deal with a redistribution of fat tissue into the lower abdomen, hips, and thighs.

Because this is reported to be the norm doesn't mean that you have to follow the pattern. Eating correctly, learning to modify behavior that results in eating to attempt to resolve stress, and exercising in an appropriate program for you can counteract the natural tendency to put on the pounds of age.

Eating Disorders

Two major types of eating disorders are bulimia nervosa and anorexia nervosa. Although they have different characteristics and manifestations, both stem from dysfunctionality in the home. The parents are often hypercritical of the child, and they discipline by using shaming techniques. Ninety-five percent of all eating disorders occur in women.

Bulimia

Bulimia is a psychologically based disorder characterized by marked shifts in weight from gain to loss. Bulimics accomplish this by bingeing and purging. This disorder can occur at any age, although signs and symptoms usually begin in the late teens. Bulimia is seen in all social groups, and 95 percent of the victims are women. In a susceptible individual, the stresses of home and personal life encourage bulimic responses. Behavior becomes increasingly secretive, isolated, and desperate. Although frequently depressed, bulimics are not allowed to reveal their feelings at home, and in turn they repress a great deal of anger.

Bulimics frequently alternate between rigid internal control and being totally out of control. Controlling activities include list making, covert rehearsal of interactions, restricted intake of food, restricted emotional expression, and rigid routines and rules. These types of behavior are a result of living in a rigidly controlling or abusive environment at home.

Out-of-control behavior includes binge eating, purging, substance abuse, binge spending, shoplifting, promiscuity, and suicide attempts. Bulimics want to control. Since they often cannot control their family members or others, bulimics learn that the only thing they can control is their appearance. So they work very diligently at trying to control their weight by bingeing or purging, depending on their emotional state at the time. Bulimia is considered an *ego dystonic behavior,* meaning the person is very distressed about her weight.

Classic symptoms of bulimia include secretive eating, bingeing, purging, caffeine abuse, low self-esteem, depression, powerlessness, obsession with appearance, menstrual disorders, dental problems, and fatigue. Bulimia may be seen as a result of the socialization process for women in Western cultures and in certain family environments. These women are often told to become one thing but see just the opposite in feminist literature. Being fragile, thin, small, and delicate is in definite conflict with being strong, powerful, and credible. If a woman gives in to the desire to overeat, she is a social failure, but if she gives in to the desire to avoid food, or purges herself, she is also considered a social failure. This conflict accentuates the eating disorder.

In my practice, I see many women with weight-control problems. The problems are not always easily recognized, and when questioned, the women frequently deny that they have any. It often requires a great deal of pain and trauma to encourage an eating-disorder patient to seek help.

Betty is such a patient. She was raised in a very well-to-do family as an only child. Her mother was a socialite, involved in all the major events in town. She had pushed—actually forced—Betty to take voice and ballet lessons and to enter talent contests and beauty pageants. Betty was disliked by other children, who felt that she was arrogant and aloof.

Weight was always an issue with Betty's mother. "Betty, if you eat that sundae, you'll never fit into your evening gown." Or, "Betty, you look as if you've gained a few pounds this week. You'd better be careful." Betty could never do quite enough to please her mother. Betty indicated to me that her father didn't seem to feel that performance was as important as her mother did, but he would not contradict her mother on these issues.

It didn't take Betty very long to realize that pleasing her mother protected her from a seething rage that could erupt at any moment. She never knew quite what it would take to please her mother. She never knew if she was dancing the right step or dancing fast enough to appease her. The best way to avoid her mother's passive-aggressiveness was to keep conflict at a minimum. By always doing things around the house for her mother and by keeping her weight down, Betty could limit the outbursts and periods of being ignored.

The ritual of bingeing and purging began to intensify when Betty was a junior in high school. She realized that she could eat what she wanted and then induce vomiting or use laxatives and keep her weight down. She felt guilty after purging but reasoned that she was avoiding her mother's wrath. When competitions or pageants were held, Betty would not eat and would purge anyway. She knew all of the makeup tricks to cover up her sunken cheeks and tired eyes.

The trophies, crowns, and prizes only partly compensated for the physical and emotional agony that she was going through. The compliments of "You're so beautiful and talented" were nice, but within her were darkness and sorrow.

Betty had determined that she would quit competing in contests when she finished high school, but a modeling agency called her mother to inquire about Betty's doing part-time work while she was in college. Once again, Mother won out, and Betty began modeling on weekends. In all their conversations with Betty, the agency representatives emphasized the need for thinness. The need to binge and purge continued.

How did Betty get to my office? Actually, her husband called me. They had married when they finished college. Now Betty was working in marketing for a large department store, and he was the manager of a restaurant.

Her husband sounded very perplexed when I talked with him on the phone.

"Dr. Hager, I just wanted to ask you a couple of questions about my wife," he said. "Is it normal for someone to get sick whenever she eats a decent-sized meal?"

"Well," I responded, "there are some digestive disorders where one might have severe indigestion or nausea after eating certain foods or large meals. Why?"

He paused and said, "I'm just worried about Betty. Whenever we go out to eat, which is often, she always comes back home, says she is sick from the food, goes into the bathroom, and vomits. Is that normal?"

"No, it isn't. You'd better make an appointment for her to see me."

I encouraged him to try to get her in as soon as possible. When Betty did come in for an exam, she was quite thin and was having only occasional light menstrual periods. I explained to her the association between percent body fat and menstrual function (see chapter 4) and encouraged appropriate nutrition. I referred her to a psychiatrist and to an eating disorders clinic. She has improved some, but as it is for most women with eating disorders, her road to recovery is long and winding.

Anorexia

Anorexia nervosa affects approximately 1 percent of adolescent and young adult women. In my practice, I am seeing more and more young women with this disorder, which, unfortunately, is very difficult to manage. The mortality rate is as high as 20 percent, usually resulting from starvation and its related metabolic effects, or from suicide.

Anorectics also come out of dysfunctional families with a social/cultural emphasis on thinness. Women with anorexia frequently give a history of extreme stress in their childhood homes. They were often pushed to do or become something that they lacked the self-esteem to accomplish. Just as stress can precipitate bingeing and purging, it can stimulate a preoccupation with weight reduction to the extent that it becomes a disease. Whereas many women respond to anxiety in their lives by eating, the anorectic responds by doing whatever is necessary to lose weight, including starving.

Women with anorexia nervosa typically have type A personalities, are perfectionistic, are easily excited, are hostile with significant repressed anger, and have accentuated cardiovascular reactions to stress. They are often very finicky and not easily satisfied with anything. Anorectics are extremely vulnerable to the mildest of stressors. They have a distorted body image, weigh less than they should, participate in eating rituals, and deny that they have a food-related problem. Anorexia is an *ego syntonic disorder*, meaning the person is proud of her emaciation.

Comparison of Anorexia and Bulimia

Anorexia Nervosa	Bulimia Nervosa
Young age of onset	Onset in late teens or early adult years
Less than minimal weight	Normal or near-normal weight
Scant or no menses	Menstrual irregularities
Distorted body image	More accurate perception of body image
Denial of food-related problems	Acknowledge abnormal eating
Appear to be in control	Impulsive
Eating rituals	Appear to eat normally when not bingeing
Only occasional vomiting	Induced vomiting, laxative abuse
Substance and sexual abuse uncommon	Substance abuse common
Frequent stress in home, often angry	Frequent stress in home, often angry, frequently victimized
Low tolerance for intimacy	Have relationships but have difficulty with intimacy
Proud of her emaciation	Distressed about her weight

Binge Eating

Binge eating disorder (BED) is a recently described problem affecting 2–3 percent of adults. It is most commonly seen with increasing degrees of weight gain. BED patients are often those who diet and stop, gain weight, and diet again. They have usually been on every diet known to woman, but have not modified their behavior to allow for consistent maintenance of weight. BED is much more common in women than in men. Weight gain and loss predisposes these women to hyperlipidemia (elevated cholesterol and triglycerides) and diabetes.

Treating Eating Disorders

As in Betty's case, stress frequently plays a role in eating disorders. Soukup published a study in which he reported that individuals with bulimia experienced more negative life events and feelings of being pressured than did individuals with no eating disorders. Eating-disorder patients reported increased levels of stress, decreased confidence in their ability to solve problems, avoidance of confronting problems, reluctance to share personal problems, and strong feelings of being driven.

Sohlberg found that the physician must tailor the therapy plan to the individual. Not all patients respond to the same forms of management. This study reported that helping patients cope with stress may reduce the damaging effects of the disorder.[2]

Laessie studied fifty-five bulimic patients and treated them with nutritional management and stress management. Both groups showed a decrease in bingeing and purging and in body dissatisfaction and depression. The quickest improvement in eating habits occurred with nutritional management and the best affect on psychological features occurred with stress management.[3]

Eating disorders require a multifaceted management approach. Techniques of stress management must be used to deal with the stress in the woman's life. Getting help from a psychologist or psychiatrist and enrolling in an eating-disorders clinic is the second step. The typical eating-disorders patient has very low self-esteem. She sees herself as one who cannot deal with life's issues and focuses on her body size as an indicator of how good she is. She must recognize that she is created in God's image, and that is the best. God sees people not merely at a surface level, but at heart level. He knows what has caused her to be the way she is and he is willing to help her make the changes necessary to redeem the damage of the past. However, she cannot go on blaming the past for all of her woes. She must determine that the dysfunction will end here. She must get into spiritual counseling and nutritional counseling. God wants her to be whole.

Eating a balanced diet, exercising, and using appropriate vitamin supplementation are the best ways to control weight. Avoid too much salt and sugar. Remember the detrimental effects caffeine and chocolate have on the system.

A Balanced Diet

Food Group	Includes	Servings Per Day
Meat	Lean meat, skinned poultry, fish, and eggs (or beans, peas, nuts)	2–3
Milk	Low-fat or skim milk, low-fat cheese, low-fat yogurt	2–4
Vegetables and Fruits	One citrus, one green or yellow vegetable, plus other fruits and vegetables	4 or more
Bread and Cereal	Whole wheat or rye bread, whole-grain cereals	4 or more
Water	Plain, in addition to any other fluids	6 glasses or more

Many people use supplemental vitamins. A well-balanced diet is the best way to get your vitamins. If you do take supplements, remember these tips:

Vitamin B1 (thiamine) in excess can cause bad breath.

Vitamin B6 (pyridoxine) in quantities of more than 200 milligrams per day may cause abnormal tingling or numbness of the extremities.

Vitamin C does not totally protect you from colds but may decrease the severity of the symptoms.

If you choose to use herbal remedies, you should make that decision in consultation with your health-care provider. Assess the benefits versus the risks of such products and seek evidence of their beneficial effects.

It Could Be Your Problem

After reading about the characteristics of bulimia, anorexia, and BED, you are probably saying, "Well, I certainly don't have any of those." That may be true, but are you at your ideal body weight? Do you respond to anxiety by eating? Does stress result in loss of appetite, diarrhea, and weight loss? If so, you probably have a weight problem and need to take steps to correct it.

Perhaps you have a friend or family member who you suspect has an eating disorder. Dr. Laura Humphreys, director of the University of Kentucky Medical School Eating Disorders Clinic, encourages these actions:

Heed the signs of the disorders.

Approach your friend gently, but persistently.

Do not discuss her eating habits.

Do focus on unhappiness as the reason she could benefit from help.

Be supportive.

Give her a written list of sources for professional help.

Don't deal with it alone.
Do talk to someone about your own emotions.[4]

Weight problems are serious because they affect so many other areas of your life. The obese person is at risk for other illnesses. There are greater risks of anesthesia and operative complications during surgery. Excessive thinness can result in menstrual disorders, as can excessive weight gain. Altered immunity, poor hygiene, poor self-esteem, and depression are all associated with altered weight. If you have a problem, get help soon. You can overcome this problem.

> Before I formed you in the womb I knew you, And before you were born I consecrated you.
>
> Jeremiah 1:5

A Spiritual Perspective

Compared to alcohol and drugs, food seems so innocuous, yet we know that extremes of weight gain or loss pose serious threats to our health and even to our lives. Can anything so potentially significant escape the interest of our heavenly Father? In 2 Corinthians 10:5, Paul implores us to take "every thought captive to the obedience of Christ" and to realize that the spiritual weapons of prayer and self-discipline have the ability to "destroy fortresses" (see v. 4). I confess that I have turned to food for comfort and to salve anger. In the end, I created a negative cycle of weight gain and self-loathing that is anything but satisfying. Over and over again, I must go back to the Lord and discuss this all with him. He tells me to forgive myself and begin anew. He woos me to himself and offers me the water that will not leave me thirsty and the food that will not leave my soul hungry.

Scriptures for Meditation

2 Corinthians 10:2–5
Matthew 4:4
Matthew 6:25–34

A Suggested Prayer

Lord, I confess that I would often rather eat some cookies than take the time to sit down and talk with you about what is really bugging me. There is too much old stuff to sort through, and eating gives me a fast fix. Food can numb my pain and replace my anger with cravings, and when I satisfy those cravings I feel better—for a little while—then it starts all over again. Help me, Lord. Help me to come to you for the long-term cure. Help me to surrender my cravings to you and to courageously deal with the feelings that are at the root of my addiction. Teach me to value wholeness more than beauty as the world defines it. Teach me to bring every thought, every desire into the captivity of constant conversation with my only true Source—you, my blessed Lord Jesus.

11

Substance Abuse

*C*hange has occurred in the roles of women in our society, changes that have been encouraged by some organizations and movements, changes that have been perceived to be necessary for survival or the attainment of certain lifestyles, changes that have been made out of a desire to achieve individual goals and dreams.

Whatever the reason for all these changes, women's lives are significantly affected by the roles they choose or feel compelled to assume. Whereas past generations of women oriented their lives around family-related goals and spent most of their working hours involved in homemaking responsibilities, many American women today are involved in some combination of paid employment and homemaking.

According to an article from the National Institute of Mental Health, 70 percent of women in the work force have children under eighteen years of age.[1] Not only are these women working outside the home, but they are grocery shopping, preparing meals, doing laundry, cleaning house, driving in car pools, and rearing children. Successfully blending and fulfilling these roles is a source of significant frustration, particularly for those who find themselves responsible for sole support, both financial and emotional, of their children. Situations such as these impose tremendous stress on women that can lead to depression and anxiety. In turn, there are temptations to look for things that will alleviate the stress, even if only temporarily. It is this search that may lead the overwhelmed woman to attempt to buffer her stress with substances.

Nan is a young woman whom I met as a patient while I was beginning to prepare the manuscript for this book. She made an appointment to see me in the office, expressing abnormal menstrual periods as her chief complaint. Though she was twenty-two years old at the time, she looked at least thirty. There was a look of emptiness in her eyes. She was nattily dressed, but her extreme thinness caused her clothes to hang on her body.

I spent the usual amount of time recording historical information about her past and current health status. She had the onset of menstrual periods at a normal time, twelve years of age. When she was sixteen, she began to skip periods occasionally. By the time she was twenty-one and a junior in college, Nan had stopped having periods altogether.

For two years this had gone on, but she never sought medical care. She admitted to having a poor appetite, weight loss, anxiety, and feeling lethargic much of the time. She was not doing well in school and was considering dropping out after the current semester.

Nan's examination was normal, except for her weight.

Before I left the exam room, I asked a question that I frequently pose in such a situation, "Nan, is there anything that is troubling you emotionally or spiritually?"

She looked at the floor, wrung her hands, and said, "I just can't talk about it today. Could I come back some other time?"

I responded with a smile and said, "Sure, you can come back anytime, just make an appointment at the front desk for a conference time."

Fearing that she would act like many young women who ask for a delay in facing the real issues in their lives and then never show up again, I added, "If you are in trouble or you aren't safe from others or yourself, we want to help you. Just let us know."

Later that day, I asked my receptionist, Dana, if Nan had made a follow-up appointment. To my great surprise, she was scheduled to return in ten days. I felt better about her safety. She had been given a prescription for progesterone to stimulate the onset of a menstrual period, and I would know the result of the treatment when she returned.

At her next appointment, she was having withdrawal bleeding from the progesterone, which meant the reason for her lack of periods was most likely the cessation of ovulation—probably a result of poor nutrition and weight loss, with decreased body fat.

I asked Nan if she would like to talk about the things that were bothering her. She started to reiterate how she was feeling now. I interrupted her and said, "Nan, would you please go back and tell me your story from the beginning?"

"Okay, I'll try," she responded. "I grew up just outside Lexington, in a small town. My father is a factory worker, and he is also an alcoholic. My mother worked part-time as a secretary. I have two brothers and a sister, and we are very close. I think never knowing when Dad was going to go on a binge and become violent kept us close, because we had to protect each other.

"Because I was afraid of being whipped by my father, I was always very obedient as a child. In fact, I don't recall doing anything really bad at all. I didn't have many friends, because the other kids were afraid of my father. He physically abused my mother but would always make up to her, and she would never say anything bad about him.

"I really wanted to have friends, so I started to hang around with a group of kids who I knew didn't have very good reputations. At least they would let me go places with them. They would even come to my house, because my dad wasn't any worse than theirs.

"All of these guys smoked, and I didn't. They kept asking me to try, and I was afraid I would get caught. Fear was always in my mind. I didn't want to lose my friends though, so I gave in and started smoking cigarettes. I was fifteen then, I think.

"Once I made the decision to smoke, it seemed that a lot of the fear I had of getting caught went away. I tried to stop a couple of times, but I would always go back because everybody else was doing it, and it made me feel good. As I look back now it seems as if that barrier being broken opened the door for the other things that followed.

"We began to go to parties a lot. There was always beer there, and a lot of the kids would smoke pot. I swore to myself that I would never drink alcohol or use drugs, because I had seen what they had done to my family. In spite of my determination, though, it was as if I just couldn't say no. I just wanted to be accepted, to be a part of what was going on. I felt that I could trust my friends to keep me from drinking too much or doing drugs.

"Soon, I was drinking pretty heavily, and I was smoking marijuana every weekend. I never studied, my grades went down, and the school counselor called my mother to see if there was a problem. They decided to have a meeting, a confrontation with me to address the problems. The counselor met with my mom, my dad, and me. I admitted that I had been smoking and that I was drinking some. I couldn't tell them about the marijuana. When my dad started criticizing me, I blew up. For the first time in my life, I yelled at him, and I ran out of the house because I was afraid the hypocrite was going to hit me.

"I wasn't eating well. I lost weight, started skipping periods, and didn't feel well. I did get my grades up some because I really did want to get into college. It just seems that once the ball started rolling downhill I couldn't stop it. After drinking all night, I would always feel horrible the next day. I started drinking harder stuff to get a high and I started spending more and more time away from home.

"A lot of the kids took prescription medication from their parents' medicine chests. We started using pain medication along with alcohol, and before I knew it I was hooked on both. About this time I began to be nauseated all the time, and I noticed that my breasts were really sore. One of the other girls had been pregnant and had the same symptoms, so she told me to go to the health department and get a pregnancy test. It was positive. I knew that my parents would be very upset, so I stole some money from my dad's money drawer and had an abortion. The guilt was unbelievable.

"The only way I knew how to handle the emotional pain was with drugs. I was doing crack by then and turning tricks to make money to support my habit. I stayed in school but was just barely getting by with my grades. I became more and more depressed about what was happening with my life. It seemed that there was no hope for anything to change. Recently, I took an overdose of downers and wound up in the emergency room after my roommate found me unconscious in our apartment. The hospital social worker arranged for me to enter a rehab program and encouraged me to see you about my periods."

I was astounded. Not by the story so much, because it is an all too frequent one, but by the candor with which this young woman recounted her life story to me, a relative stranger.

"Nan, I'm so glad you came back. I was afraid you wouldn't. I know it isn't easy to talk about the sadness in your life, but that is the first step in getting well."

"Yeah, I know," she replied. "I learned that at Alcoholics Anonymous."

Stress and Addiction

The use of substances to attempt to handle stress is an all too common event in the lives of women and men. You may recall from the opening chapter in this book that stress can result in the release of epinephrine and norepinephrine from the adrenal glands. The initial release of these chemicals may result in a pleasurable feeling of being in control of the stress. Similarly, nicotine, caffeine, alcohol, and some drugs can result in the same feelings. Alcohol and narcotics quickly become depressants, however. These substances, which are used as stress buffers to reduce the awareness of ongoing stressful life events, are really temporizing in their effects and subsequently introduce new stresses that overwhelm the individual and promote the continued use of more stress buffers. The snowball rolling downhill that Nan described begins to cause its devastating effects.

The perception of the person addicted to substances is that the chemical enables her to cope with daily stresses. The addictive cycle begins. This is especially true in the person who has inherited an addictive personality. Although a careful family history can frequently reveal a tendency toward this behavior, it is often unknown by the individual until she begins to use the substance.

Nan exemplifies a tendency that has been eloquently described by Dr. Richard Clayton at the University of Kentucky. He has found that there is a progression in the drug addict from use of socially acceptable substances to socially unacceptable drugs. Most people start the process with nicotine, move on to beer and wine, to harder alcohol, to marijuana, and finally to hard drugs. The progression does not always go as far as street drugs, but once initiated, the potential exists.

Caffeine

I want to begin this section on specific substances by mentioning a very socially acceptable substance to which I was addicted until five years ago. When I was enlisted in the U.S. Public Health Service, assigned to the Centers for Disease Control, I became addicted to caffeine. We had frequent meetings. I spent a great deal of time writing and doing research. It was easy to grab a cup of coffee early in the morning and keep refilling it all day. Before long, I found that I had to have coffee to start the day, to get through the day, and even to end the day. I was averaging twelve to fourteen cups. Coffee didn't affect my sleep. I could go to sleep right after drinking a cup. When I couldn't get coffee, I would become agitated and shaky and I would get a headache. What did I do to relieve the symptoms? Drink more coffee. This same pattern is seen in those who find themselves addicted to any drug. Initiation of the habit is innocent; the effects of addiction are devastating.

When I returned to the practice of obstetrics and gynecology and to teaching, I did not have the time to ingest the same amount of caffeine. I experienced withdrawal symptoms. I decided that I did not want to be addicted to anything, so I quit cold turkey. The symptoms were horrible for about three weeks, but they did resolve. Now I have no desire for caffeine at all. I feel better physically and emotionally because I'm not hooked on a substance.

Caffeine triggers the release of adrenaline from the adrenal glands. Each cup of coffee, with its 125 milligrams of caffeine, acts as a stimulant. The feeling of control over stress is actually overcome rapidly by an aggravation of stress, because you are chronically stimulated and you begin to overrespond to stress.

Caffeine causes constriction of blood vessels, which can affect the heart and the vascular system. Heart patients and hypertensive patients should not use caffeine. Caffeine use can also have damaging effects on the vascular system in pregnancy. Heavy drinkers of caffeine can get severe headaches as a result of vascular spasm if they go eighteen to twenty-four hours without the substance. Remember, from chapter 5, that caffeine can often relieve a migraine sufferer's headache and may be used occasionally for acute relief. Moderate to heavy users of caffeine can also develop insomnia, anxiety, and gastric ulcers.

Nicotine

Nicotine, like caffeine, is seldom considered by the public to be a drug. Most people feel that they can control their caffeine intake and their use of nicotine—an amazing statement when you consider that fifty million Americans smoke, and 98 percent of these are addicted to nicotine. One-third to one-half of smokers will die nicotine-related deaths from diseases such as lung cancer and heart disease. The tar from cigarettes has a definite carcinogenic effect on the lungs, and nicotine and carbon monoxide adversely affect the function of the lungs and heart.

The rates of lung cancer in women are increasing due primarily to a rapidly increasing prevalence of cigarette smoking in females. Lung cancer is the second leading cause of cancer death among women. The carcinogenic dose of nicotine is estimated to be one pack per day, smoking for seventeen years. (This is the equivalent of 125,000 cigarettes.) Ninety-one percent of people who are found to have lung cancer die within five years of the time their diagnosis is made.

Because nicotine is an addictive drug, many women who want to quit find that they cannot. In addition, the use of nicotine is often the first step along the pathway to the use of harder drugs. The best way to avoid the progression to addiction is to avoid smoking or to stop if you smoke now.

I would remind you that you cannot do it alone, in most situations, and will need the help of a quit-smoking program and possibly a medical aid such as nicotine patches. Remember that if you smoked regularly and heavily, it will take twelve years to rid your body of the residue of tars and nicotine.

The tobacco companies know that nicotine is addictive. If they can get young people to try smoking, they have an excellent chance of hooking them into the habit for a lifetime. We must caution young women not to smoke their first cigarette.

Alcohol

The use of alcohol is very socially acceptable behavior by men and women of this country and many other nations. Some religions, some Protestant denominations, and some sects condemn the use of any alcohol, yet in surveys the majority of Americans indicate that controlled use is acceptable and will not cause problems.

The variable in that statement is *controlled.* Many individuals do not know whether they can control their drinking at the time of their first ingestion of alcohol. Alcohol abuse affects one in three American families. In the United States, 13.8 percent of Americans have an alcohol-use problem at some time in their lives, with a male to female ratio of five to one.

There is strong evidence of a genetic predisposition to addictive behavior of all sorts and equally good evidence of a predisposition to alcohol abuse. If the individual takes that first drink, and she has inherited the predisposition to an addictive personality, it may be the first step to alcoholism. Many would say that responsible drinking can be taught to children and adolescents, but if the persons doing the teaching are not responsible themselves, the children will not be able to distinguish between the lesson and the example. In addition, the stresses of life may be different for that child, and the desire to overcome the effects of stress by drinking may be too great to resist.

Nan is a classic example of one who saw the damaging effects of alcohol in her own home yet could not resist the temptation when it came, and once she started, she could not stop.

Stress affects different people in different ways, regarding its stimulation to use and abuse substances. Stress does not appear to play as significant a role in the ingestion of alcohol in women as it does in men. Data from the Health and Nutrition Examination Survey indicate that stress does appear to play a role in the control of alcohol ingestion by adolescents.[2]

Alcohol affects psychological stress through its ability, in conjunction with ongoing activity, to affect the amount of attention paid to stressful thoughts. Regular drinkers use alcohol to dissipate the stress and worry of vocation, financial problems, and relational and marital problems. Many drinkers use alcohol to help them feel socially accepted. Nan admitted this. The effects of alcohol on the central nervous system diminish the boundaries of restraint and make the drinker feel more secure.

There are several biochemical mechanisms in the central nervous system that contribute to craving of alcohol in problem drinkers. Studies have shown an increase in the intake of alcohol when subjects were fed nutrient-deficient diets, when they had low blood sugars (hypoglycemia), or when they were placed in stressful environments.

Alcohol intake is not without its benefits. The old saying goes, "You never see a wino die of a heart attack." Drinking up to two ounces (two drinks) of alcohol a day has been associated with increases in high-density lipoprotein (HDL) or "good" cholesterol. It has also been associated with longevity. The problem is that many drinkers do not or cannot limit their intake to two drinks a day, and the reliance and dependence on alcohol grows.

The hazards of alcohol include effects on the endocrine system, the heart, the liver, the bone marrow, and the reproductive system. Alcohol stimulates the release of cortisol from the adrenal glands, which promotes the retention of sodium and the loss of potassium. Sodium retention can result in elevation of the blood pressure, although this is often counteracted by the diuretic (fluid-losing) effects. Potassium loss in sufficient amounts can make the heart vulnerable to abnormal rhythms. Alcohol can also cause direct damage to the heart muscle, making it flabby and lax, with decreased pumping capability.

Alcohol is broken down—metabolized—in the liver. Excessive intake stresses the capacity of the liver and cirrhosis (enlargement and hardening) can result. Dilated veins—varices—may form in the esophagus when the veins in the liver become plugged, and new veins form to bypass the obstructed organ. These varices can rupture and bleed. Alcohol can also have a direct effect on the bone marrow, decreasing its ability to make red blood cells.

Unique Effects of Alcoholism in Women

1. Women advance more rapidly than men from the onset of problem drinking to the development of adverse medical consequences.
2. Women metabolize alcohol more slowly than men.
3. Women are statistically more likely to develop cirrhosis of the liver.
4. Women have more frequent concurrent mood, anxiety, eating, and psychosexual disorders than men.
5. Women are at greater risk for death than male alcoholics.
6. Women seek addiction therapy less frequently than men.

Some effects of alcohol are seen more frequently in women than in men. Women metabolize alcohol more slowly than men do and can become intoxicated on smaller volumes of alcohol than can men. Possible reasons include a smaller total blood volume for distribution of alcohol in the body, since women are generally smaller; a lower rate of metabolism by the lining of the stomach; and influences of estrogen.

Women have been found to advance more rapidly than men from the initial onset of problem drinking to the development of adverse medical consequences. This places women alcoholics at a greater risk for death than male alcoholics. Smith followed alcoholics over time and found that 31 percent of women were dead at an eleven-year follow-up. This was four times as many deaths as expected for women in the general population. Statistically women are also more likely to develop cirrhosis of the liver.

Females who are problem drinkers have been found to have more concurrent mood, anxiety, eating, and psychosexual disorders than men. Studies indicate that these women often have very low self-esteem. They are frequently poorly nourished, abuse other substances, and have a history of sexual abuse.

Alcoholism can affect reproductive function in both sexes. In women, there is an association with absence of menstrual periods, absence of ovulation, inadequate production of progesterone in the latter part of the menstrual cycle, increased risks of miscarriage, and early onset of menopause. The offspring of women who drink heavily during pregnancy may have fetal alcohol syndrome, including birth defects.

The final point of difference between female and male alcoholics is perhaps the most damaging. Studies indicate that alcohol-dependent women seek treatment for their addiction less frequently than men do. This may be because there is a perception that alcohol use is less socially acceptable for women or that programs are more geared toward men. If your answer to any of the following four questions is yes, you should seek help for your dependence on alcohol.

Alcohol-Dependence Indicators

Have you made repeated attempts to cut down on your drinking?
Do you get angry if anyone asks about your drinking?
Do you feel guilty about your drinking?
Do you use an "eye opener" drink in the morning to calm your nerves?

Drugs

It is beyond the scope of this book to discuss drug addiction in detail. Many good books and programs for addiction are offered; unfortunately the cure rates are quite variable.

Numerous prescription medications can result in dependence when they are used repeatedly or excessively. To avoid untoward interactions, make your physician aware of all the medications you are taking. Do not persist in seeking potentially addictive medications if your physician has told you not to use them.

Tranquilizers are used to decrease anxiety and tension. Occasionally, these medications are necessary on a temporary basis to relieve acute stress. You can develop a psychological dependence for such medications very easily. The more you use, the more you feel you need. The key is to find the cause for your anxiety and deal with it directly.

Amphetamines (uppers) cause the release of adrenaline into the system. They are frequently an ingredient in weight-loss pills. Users of such drugs to elevate mood or for weight reduction develop a dependence on the medication. When they stop using amphetamines, there is a rebound effect, and the lethargy and/or increased appetite return. That is why diet pills only work temporarily.

Sleeping pills act on the central nervous system to promote sleep. Occasionally you may have to take a pill to enable you to get much needed sleep in a stressful situation, but dependence can easily develop when they are used repeatedly. Chronic use can lead to lethargy and lassitude. The key to proper sleep is resolution of anxiety and stress, proper diet and exercise, and learning to relax.

Analgesics are medications used to relieve pain. Pain thresholds differ significantly among individuals. At times, pain relief is necessary when injury or surgery occur. Unfortunately, many people use analgesics for minor aches and pains as well. The feelings of well-being and relaxation that occur are temporary, so the person repeats the dose to perpetuate the sensation. Great care must be used to avoid becoming physiologically addicted, because it will take more and more to get the same effect, and the next step will be harder drugs.

Substance abuse has many consequences. Nan experienced several of them, but abusers may experience others: physical illness and lack of well-being; poor nutrition and weight loss; increased rates of long-term depression; lack of ability to focus on goals and accomplish them; failed interpersonal relationships, frequently with breakups of marriages; excessive guilt; and loss of self-esteem.

Nan sought care. Although she didn't come in for help for substance abuse, we were able to identify the problem and encourage her to get involved with a rehabilitation program. She has started on the difficult, lengthy path to recovery.

Obviously the best way to avoid addiction to substances is to never experiment with their use, since you truly do not know if you have an addictive personality. Resolution of stress by use of the techniques mentioned later in the book will help alleviate your need to use substances to accomplish the same thing. Be assured, substances are only a temporary measure. Recognition that you are only whole and complete in your relationship with God is essential.

> Now the deeds of the flesh are evident, which are: immorality, impurity, sensuality, idolatry, sorcery, enmities, strife, jealousy, outbursts of anger, disputes, dissensions, factions, envying, drunkenness, carousing, and things like these, of which I forewarn you just as I have forewarned you that those who practice such things shall not inherit the kingdom of God.
>
> Galatians 5:19–21

A Spiritual Perspective

Addictions are Satan's counterfeit offer of wholeness and completion. Knowing our propensity for fast fixes, he offers us substances that really work—for a little while. By the time we realize the diminishing returns we receive from our chosen substance, a habit has been formed, and Satan has us right where he wants us.

The recognition of wholeness and completion that are the essence of a right relationship with God comes as a process, over time. We build a history with the Lord as we choose to spend time with him. We begin to be more willing to rely on him as we are able to choose obedience in the face of fear and doubt. Someone has said, "Feel the fear and do it scared." The lyrics of an old hymn warn us, "If we tarry till we're ready, we will never come at all." Remember that God loves you right where you are, but he cares about you too much to leave you there.

Scriptures for Meditation

> Jeremiah 29:13–14; 31:13
> Romans 3:23; 8:1
> 1 John 1:5–10
>
> These Scripture passages are designed to make a scriptural case for self-forgiveness. Read them and see for yourself how God views sin and forgiveness.

A Suggested Prayer

God, I have trouble believing that you love me just as I am. I disgust myself, so why not you? I know you created me with more in mind than this endless cycle of addiction that I have fallen into. I want out, but I am afraid to put away these things with their awful power to relieve my pain, however temporarily. I am choosing to believe that you will always be merciful. I am feeling the fear and coming to you scared. Do not forsake me, dear God. Hold fast to me until I can hold, by the strength of my will, to you.

12

Skin Disorders

"David, what do you think this is on my leg?" Linda asked as I walked into our den one evening. She pulled up the leg of her sweat suit and removed the sock from her left foot. When Linda had elevated her leg onto the stool, I could see an angry red, thick-appearing, round eruption of the skin just above the left ankle. "It itches all the time, especially at night. Sometimes when I awaken in the morning it's bleeding where I have scratched it in my sleep."

"How long has it been there?" I asked.

"Well, it started about three months ago, and it seems to come and go but never completely clears up," Linda replied. "When it improves, the skin becomes very thick and hardened."

"Do you have any other skin disorders?" I questioned. I knew that she didn't but merely wanted her to confirm my impression.

"No, but I did have a small irritated area in this same spot last year when Daddy died."

Linda had been under a lot of stress recently. Her mother was ill with metastatic breast cancer. Linda had enrolled in graduate school, intending to get a master's in biblical studies. Her duties on a church committee had become hectic and difficult, and her chronic sacroiliac problem had flared up, causing intense pain. As I reflected on all these stresses, I wondered if they could play any role in this irritating skin disorder.

I thought about my patients with similar complaints. Although the disorder is not frequent, I recalled several women who had told me about intermittent flare-ups of localized, reddened, scaly patches that seemed to recur in association with periods of stress. I had researched the literature and discovered that the association of emotional factors and stress with skin disorders has been recognized for years. The name of the disorder is *neurodermatitis*, or to be more correct medically, *lichen simplex chronicus*.

"I really think you should see a dermatologist to be sure, Linda, but the fact that you associate this skin eruption with stressful times in your life and the fact that it is a circumscribed, scaly patch that itches makes me think it is probably neurodermatitis," I stated, feeling proud that I could diagnose something that was not obstetrics-gynecology related.

According to Koo, three categories of skin disorders are associated with emotional factors and stress.[1]

1. There are skin diseases in which the severity of the condition is influenced by emotions.
2. There are disorders in which skin conditions are self-induced.
3. There are psychological problems resulting from disfiguring skin conditions.

Neurodermatitis, a condition that is classified under the group of disorders called eczema, falls under category 1. It is characterized by circumscribed, scaly patches of thickened, reddish skin that cause intense itching. The itching is so intense that the patient often rubs the area raw (this is called *excoriation*).

The incidence of this disorder is not known, but it is not infrequent, especially among women who are seen for counseling. The clinical appearance of the lesions is quite characteristic.

There is usually a single recurrent area of involvement, but in certain cases, these may be multiple. The most common areas to find eruptions of neurodermatitis are those that are subject to minor irritations and are easily reached to scratch. They may easily be confused with psoriasis because they are similarly thickened and scaly.

Common sites of involvement include the back of the head above the neck, the face, hands, wrists, forearms, elbows, thighs, lower legs, and feet. The ankles are frequently involved, and because they are easily scratched with the other foot, become angry red and quite thickened. Anal and vulvar involvement may occur and is difficult to distinguish from other skin disorders that occur in those areas.

Clinically, the areas of involvement are found to have very sharp margins. The marked redness and blisters that are seen with classic eczema are not seen with neurodermatitis. The skin is usually thickened. Small raised bumps, called papules, may occur in a pattern or be separate and raised. Scratching of these sites may contaminate them with bacteria and result in infection, causing even more redness and warmth.

A variant of this skin disorder is called polymorphic neurodermatitis. With this condition, varying types of lesions occur at the same or different times. They will vary in their extensiveness, how long they last, and their appearance.

Polymorphic neurodermatitis goes through two phases. In the first, there are draining, weeping, round or oval patches. In the second phase, these weeping lesions regress and become dry. Scars may occur at these sites when they scab over. Psychosomatic factors are frequently present in women with polymorphic neurodermatitis.

A condition similar to neurodermatitis may occur on the vulva (the lips outside the vagina). The vulva, or labia, become thickened and dry, and increased whitish pigmentation may occur. There is severe, chronic itching. Psychologic factors may contribute to its development and persistence. Effectively dealing with the stress that exacerbates the condition can help in resolving the itching. A biopsy of the vulva may be necessary to ensure that the woman does not have a cancer.

Treatment Options

The treatment of neurodermatitis varies with the individual because the underlying cause may vary. Two things are crucial in therapy. First, scratching must be prevented. If the area of involvement is not continually scratched and irritated, it will resolve. Medications like Benadryl may be used to accomplish this. Second, the underlying stress or psychiatric disorder must be evaluated and managed. If there is underlying depression, mania, obsessive-compulsive behavior, or anxiety, it should be treated with appropriate behavioral therapy or psychotherapy. Medication may be required, but in many cases, resolving stress is the key to improvement.

The area of involvement on the skin is best treated with a steroid cream. Many different preparations exist, and your dermatologist or family physician can prescribe one for you. On the vulva, we initiate treatment with a nonfluorinated steroid cream and then change to hydrocortisone cream.

Women with vulvar dermatitis should avoid bubble baths, bath salts, douching, feminine hygiene sprays, powders, and scented pads. If the itching does not resolve with steroid creams, then an antihistamine may be prescribed at night to help relieve the scratching and allow the area time to heal.

When stress recurs, it is not unusual for the patch of neurodermatitis to develop again. The itching and scratching start all over, and the patient is miserable until the process can be treated and the stress resolved. In some situations, recurrent episodes of neurodermatitis will occur over several years and then abate forever or for many years.

Linda did see a dermatologist, and the diagnosis was neurodermatitis. The area of skin breakdown and itching did not resolve immediately, just as the stressful issues did not vanish right away. She was treated with hydrocortisone cream. Slowly the ring-shaped area decreased in size. The redness began to fade into pallor, and healthy skin covered the previously scaly circle. She had several flare-ups of the disorder in the same location over a two-year period of time, but has had none since.

All red, scaly skin eruptions that itch are not a result of neurodermatitis. If these symptoms sound familiar to you though, be sure that the diagnosis is considered when you are evaluated by your physician.

> And do not seek what you shall eat, and what you shall drink, and do not keep worrying. For all these things the nations of the world eagerly seek; but your Father knows that you need these things. But seek for His kingdom, and these things shall be added to you.
>
> Luke 12:29–31

A Spiritual Perspective

"Well, you've gone too far now," you say. "I can believe that stress in my life can contribute to the occurrence of these other disorders, but rashes and skin lesions—come on now."

Yes, stress can manifest in many ways, even in disorders of the skin. In the days of Jesus, leprosy was a prevalent disease that resulted in damage to the skin. One of the principal reasons that the skin was damaged and fingers and toes were missing was the effect of leprosy on the nerve endings. The lack of sensitivity in the nerves prevented the person from feeling pain appropriately. Therefore a leper might put his hand in fire and not know it or step on a nail and not feel it. The disease was internal, but the effects were external.

It is much the same in our lives. The disarray inside results in changes that occur externally, so we focus our diagnostic and therapeutic energies on the obvious, when we really need to effect an internal cure. Jesus always had concern for the root of the problem at heart level, even when he was healing the external disease.

In the Old Testament, there is an elaborate description of the offering that lepers were to make when they were cleansed of their disease. Two birds were to be presented: One was killed and the other released. The bird that was killed symbolized purification; the one that was released was a symbol of the person's newfound freedom from disease. Has the stress in your life been resolved by the touch of the Master so that you can celebrate in your newfound joy?

Scriptures for Meditation

> Luke 11:39–44
> 2 Corinthians 4:17–18
> These Scriptures emphasize the importance of the unseen. The unseen can be most powerful!
> What unseen pressures are at work in your life now? Can you tie the onset of your skin disorder to the entry of some new source of tension that has come into your life?

A Suggested Prayer

O God, Creator of my body, I am tired of the things in my life that burden me so and result in consequences that affect my health and my soul. Please show me ways to resolve the stress that I face, and do a cleansing work in my heart so that I can celebrate in a newfound freedom.

13

Affairs

*T*he ramifications of stress are far reaching. While information in this book documents the many ways it can affect physical well-being, stress can also have a major impact on emotional, psychological wholeness.

One of the ways to deal with the crunch of all this stress is to look for an outlet. Some women look for someone for whom they don't have to be provider, wife, or mother. The end result of their search may be an affair.

Tanya, a twenty-nine-year-old woman, has been a patient of mine since she became engaged to Randy. They were married when he finished college and he assumed the day-to-day management of his father's construction company. The housing market was good, and Randy's company was a major force in the home-building business. They specialized in executive homes and built some gorgeous houses.

Tanya finished college a year after Randy graduated. Although the construction business was good, the young couple felt that having two salaries would help them to begin to accomplish some of their early financial goals. Tanya found employment as a computer programmer with a local firm. She worked for two years and enjoyed the feeling of helping to provide income that they would save to eventually build their own dream home.

Randy worked long hours, and there were many late meals at nine or ten o'clock. Tanya didn't particularly like waiting up for a worn-out husband, but she did manage to get some housework done, and they spent quality time together on weekends and vacations. During one of those times away, Tanya forgot her birth-control pills. They figured that they would be safe for a week, but as you might guess, no such luck. Tanya conceived. Their feelings were mixed about a pregnancy at this time, but they decided that it wasn't such a bad time to start a family. Tanya would work until she delivered and then stay home to care for their baby.

Tanya was a bubbly, energetic young woman who was like a little girl who just found her first doll under the Christmas tree. She was thrilled to be pregnant. "I can't ever remember being happier," she told me. "This will be so great for Randy and me. I really think it will bring us closer as a couple."

Tanya delivered a healthy baby boy, with no complications. She nursed the little guy, and he obviously thrived on the breast milk, weighing twenty-two pounds at six months of age. Tanya weaned Daniel at nine months. To her surprise, within a few months she was pregnant again. This time the pregnancy was not as exciting. When she came for her prenatal visits, Tanya was always tired. She carried Daniel on her right hip as her abdomen became more and more protuberant. The nausea abated, but the swelling of the feet and hands and the constant pressure on the diaphragm soon followed. By the time baby Jessica was born, Tanya was saying, "I don't ever want to be pregnant again, Randy. You can have the next baby yourself."

She and Randy had a long discussion about their future. His working hours were getting even longer now that his father had retired. Tanya was exasperated by the never-ending responsibilities of being a mother and wife. A twenty-two-month-old got into everything, and a newborn demanded constant attention. Randy helped when he could, but he just wasn't there very much.

When she came in for an office visit, I counseled Tanya about what men are like. "Tanya, sometimes you have to be very specific when you talk to us," I explained. "I should have known better myself, but I wasn't as supportive of my wife as I should have been when she was pregnant. It is so easy for us to get caught up in our work and the desire to provide for our families that we don't nurture our relationships with our wives. Tell Randy what is troubling you. Tell him that you need time together, time alone to be totally present to each other."

The next time I saw Tanya was one year later. She had made an appointment for a conference and an examination. I could tell that she was troubled. I recalled the bubbly, pregnant young woman who had appeared in my office several years ago, so excited about her future. Now she was obviously distraught and anxious. "Tanya, tell me, what is going on in your life?" I inquired.

"Dr. Hager, I'm so embarrassed, I didn't think I could tell you, but I have to talk with someone that I trust," she said, choking back the tears. "You know how controlling Randy is and how he thinks it is all right for him to be out late working, but I have to be home caring for the kids and keeping house. He just never seems to understand how much work that is. He loves the children, but he just doesn't spend the time with them that they need from their father. He—"

"Wait a minute, Tanya," I interrupted. "You're telling me secondhand all of this stuff about Randy. Tell me about yourself. What is going on with you?"

She began to cry softly and then burst into sobs. It was almost five minutes before she could regain her composure and speak again. I had moved to a chair near hers and offered a Kleenex.

"I went back to work last year because I was just going crazy at home with the kids. We decided to put them into day care. Fortunately, I was able to get my old job back. I would get the children ready in the morning, take them to the day care center, work eight hours, pick them up, and go home to fix dinner. Sometimes Randy would get home to eat with us, but usually he came home after Daniel and Jessica were in bed. We were both so tired that we didn't have the energy to talk, much less have sex. Sometimes weeks would go by when we wouldn't have intercourse. I felt empty, disconnected, and unloved."

"Tanya, you know what the fundamental problem is, don't you?" I asked.

"You didn't let me finish," she blurted out. "There's more.

"I've always gotten along well with my boss. He's very understanding and a great listener. He could tell that I wasn't myself and asked if he could do anything to help. We would talk a lot, and I began to tell him about Randy and the children and all of the stresses I was facing. I even told him that we never had time for sex anymore. My boss and I would go out for lunch and just talk. It was great to have someone who was interested in me and my problems. He was genuinely interested in what was bothering me and would give me advice about how to handle various situations.

"Dr. Hager, he's married and has a family. We were just friends, talking and enjoying each other's company. One day, he asked me to come with him to his house to pick up some papers he had forgotten. I went in with him. Just inside the doorway to the entrance hall, he put his arms around me and kissed me. It felt so good to be held and kissed by someone I had connected with emotionally. I kissed him back. Before we knew it, we were in his bedroom, and we were making love.

"I felt so guilty that I left work early. I was embarrassed when I picked up the kids, because I felt that everybody was looking at me. I fed the children and went to bed early so I wouldn't have to talk to Randy.

"I swore that it wouldn't happen again, but things didn't get better at home, and I needed to be loved so much that it did happen again and again and again. I really loved him and thought he loved only me. I should have known that if he did this with me he must have done it with someone else. Now I've developed warts on the outside of my vagina. I'm scared. What if I have AIDS?"

Tanya's examination did confirm genital warts caused by human papilloma virus, one of the most prevalent sexually transmitted diseases in the United States today.

I asked her if she really wanted her marriage with Randy to continue, and she responded affirmatively. I emphasized how important it was to end the relationship with her boss, get into counseling along with Randy, confess to him what had been going on, and indicate her desire to make a go of their marriage. I assured her that I would talk to the marriage counselor about Randy's role in this situation, since it was obvious that he had major changes to make if the marriage was to survive.

Stories like Tanya and Randy's are being played out daily all across America. White, Black, Hispanic; Catholic, Jew, Protestant; rich or poor; churched or unchurched—it doesn't matter. We are all potentially susceptible to the temptation to seek relief from our marital stresses in other relationships.

With two-thirds of all wives in the work force trying to be providers, mothers, and wives, is it any wonder that there is little time left for their marriages to be nurtured? If couples choose to have both husband and wife employed outside the home, then husbands must be willing to help at home with child rearing and homemaking. If not, they may find themselves playing out a Tanya-Randy scenario.

The Cost of Two Incomes

I do not deny the necessity of a husband and wife working in order to have enough income to purchase the things they desire, but at what cost to their family, especially their children? We are beginning to see the consequences of no mothers in the home. Violent crime, substance abuse, teenage pregnancy, and sexually transmitted diseases are all seen in increasing frequency. The responsibility does not just belong to women, but to all of us for our greed.

The demands made by small children, the pressures of a job outside the home, as well as demands to keep meals prepared, clothes washed and ironed, and the house cleaned create isolation from adult companionship. A woman may begin to feel that she doesn't communicate with people on an adult intellectual level. There is less and less time for family. Friends get crowded out too. She may begin to hunger for companionship, support, understanding, communication, touching, and love.

She may be unaware of how tired and run down she is. She begins to think that being lethargic is the normal way to feel. She may also begin to become angry—an underlying, seething type of anger, because she feels victimized by all of her responsibilities. This is accentuated if her spouse—or if she is single, her friends—do not appreciate what she is going through and do not offer support.

She may also be unaware of how much she longs for true intimacy. She longs to connect conversationally and emotionally; she longs to have leisure time with her husband and to experience the passion of sexual intimacy at a time other than when she is in bed and worn out at the end of a long day. The bonding of sexual intimacy doesn't occur at home, and she becomes a prime target for an affair, even if she could not imagine that ever happening.

It is important to remember that lack of sexual interest in her husband is not the problem. It is a symptom of an underlying problem—a problem that is not solved, but made worse, by an affair.

Often we need to do the changing rather than trying to change our spouses. I was guilty of this in the early days of my marriage. Whenever we faced a problem in our marriage, I would immediately focus on Linda's role in the situation, blaming her. It takes insight and maturity to admit that I am wrong and the source of the problem. The easiest thing to do is to blame someone else, and who is closer than my spouse? In not admitting my own faults and taking the initiative to change, I constantly waited for some transformation in my wife, even when she had no reason to change. When things continued as they always had, I became more angry at her, and the schism between us grew wider.

Fortunately, I was brought to my senses when things deteriorated and our marriage was on the brink of collapse. I had to acknowledge my own shortcomings and determine that I was willing to change. Counseling and spiritual direction were necessary for me to see my brokenness. Surprisingly, as I began to change, I was amazed at the changes that occurred in Linda.

An affair may seem to offer relief from the stresses you face and might look as if it will restore the feelings you have missed for so long. Instead of short-term escape, the result is long-term stress as you begin to live a double life at home. You know that it isn't right, but you cannot break away and leave the way you feel in the other man's arms.

I am not condoning a double standard here. Men are susceptible to the same temptations. We want to be appreciated for what we do to provide for our families. We want to be understood, even though we have to struggle to be open, sharing, and conversant people. If we don't find fulfillment in our marriages, we may be irrational and assume that things will be better in someone else's bed.

We must work to prevent the conditions that create an ideal environment for an affair. Stress reduction and time management are important, but if we don't use the extra time to invest in emotional and spiritual development and in our marriages and families, it will be more time wasted. Quality and quantity time together is essential. We must share responsibility in our work outside and inside the home. Communication must be open and honest. We must show our mates that we value them, and pursue them as though we were dating again, doing the loving, thoughtful things we did back then. We must pray and study God's Word together. Then our marriages will be more affair proof, and we will love each other in a way that will negate our need for another intimate relationship.

Appraise your real spiritual, emotional, and relational needs as opposed to your perceived material needs, and make important decisions that will emphasize a commitment to God first, spouse and family second, and yourself and career appropriately third. It is sad that in striving to attain what feminist leaders have preached as equality with men, many women have sacrificed their own physical and emotional well-being.

Tanya and Randy have been in marriage counseling for over a year. I have been pleasantly surprised at his willingness to change for the benefit of his wife and family. He has hired someone to assist in his administrative responsibilities and is taking time off to be with Tanya and the children.

Tanya confessed her role in the marital disharmony and instead of finding anger and resentment, as she expected, found love and forgiveness. She confronted her boss with her determination to end the affair and quit her job as a computer programmer. She is working part-time for another company and is pleased with the changes in her life.

> For their heart was not steadfast toward Him,
> Nor were they faithful in His covenant.

But He, being compassionate, forgave their iniquity, and
did not destroy them.

Psalm 78:37–38

A Spiritual Perspective

When I was a little girl, I forgot what my father looked
like. His career as a preacher and evangelist took him all
over the world, and consequently he was never in my little world for very long. Now he is in heaven, yet I still look
for his face.

All my life, I will have to pray against the temptation
to find my father in other men. All my life, I will be hungry for the intimacy with my father that I never experienced but always longed for. Until I was able to own this
fact, I made some unwise choices in relationships.
Sometimes I advertised something I did not really have
for sale. My life and health could have been wrecked by
this desire.

Even writing this down causes me discomfort and
shame. I don't like this hunger within and what it has
threatened to do to me, but I cannot escape its truth.
When the emptiness of fatherlessness becomes too
strong, I go to my heavenly Father. I know my earthly father would say to me: "Don't wreck your life because of
the things I failed to do. Trust our Father." I know my heavenly Father loves me more than any earthly man ever
could, and I am learning to rest in this knowledge.

Scriptures for Meditation

Psalm 103
Isaiah 54:4–5

The Scriptures plainly state that God wants to meet our very deepest need for intimacy. The need for satisfying intimacy is inherent to the human condition. There is no shame in that desire, but Satan loves to offer us counterfeits. Why? Because he knows that if he can deceive us into believing that our need for intimacy can be fully satisfied by the physical act of sex, he will have led us to a path that ultimately ends in total self-destruction and death.

How are you meeting your deep need for intimacy?

Suggested Spiritual Exercise

Close your eyes and rest. Picture Jesus coming into the room. He walks over to you and folds you gently into his arms. He tousles your hair and kisses you gently on the cheek. He takes your face into his hands and looks deeply into your eyes. No words are necessary as you communicate soul to soul. Believe he loves you as he loves no one else on earth. You are a unique creation of the Father, and no one can take your place with him. Receive this love that will go with you through even the valley of the shadow of death. Let this love begin to heal you from the inside out.

14

Stress Resolution Guidelines

*A*fter reading this far, you are aware of the physical, emotional, and spiritual consequences of unmanaged stress in the lives of women. However, women do not have to suffer its consequences. By using techniques for stress management, taking care of themselves physically and emotionally, and utilizing spiritual resources, they can be survivors not overcome by stress. I have witnessed this triumph in the lives of many of my patients.

Is it abnormal to have stress in your life? Obviously not. Various amounts of stress are present in all our lives. We can't avoid it. Stressful events can be negative, such as rejection in a relationship, loss of a job, or financial pressures; stressful events can be positive, like the challenge of an exam, receiving a longed-for promotion at work, or buying a new home. A normal amount of stress is called *eustress*. Too much stress is called *distress*. We need eustress to encourage growth, maturity, alertness, and improvement in our lives. Stress encourages problem-solving and forces us to either face challenges and overcome them or crumble beneath their steamroller effect.

Keeping in mind the following facts may help you better cope with the stressful situation(s) you confront:

1. Stress is a fact of life that may have either positive or negative consequences.
2. Stress reactions are unique to the individual—what is stressful to one person may not be stressful to another.
3. To a large degree, your perceptions determine what is stressful to you.
4. Effective stress management requires understanding how stress affects you.
5. Managing stress effectively is a learned skill requiring time, trial, and determination.
6. You need to identify enjoyable activities, both physical and mental, that help you dissipate stress.
7. Any chronic, unresolved condition should be evaluated by a health-care professional and may require medical treatment.

When you understand these facts, you need to consider certain self-help techniques to assist in the dissipation of stress.

The first step in stress management is recognizing that you are stressed. Often I see patients who are obviously stressed to the max but deny that it is affecting them. You must acknowledge the problem in order to solve it.

Another key step in stress management is to understand how stress affects you. How do you react to stress? Has stress so affected you that you have one of the diseases described in these chapters? Then you may benefit from learning to manage your stress more effectively. Stress depends on your perception of what is stressful, the situation in which you find yourself, and how you have learned to react. Because these conditions vary with the individual, no one can write a universal prescription for coping. However, there are some basic stress-management principles and self-help techniques that have been described by various experts.

Techniques to Reduce Stress

Learn to relax
Practice acceptance
Evaluate your situation
Get organized
Talk to friends
Exercise
Eat right
Watch your habits
Have quiet time
Embark on a journey with God

I believe that being on a journey with God and allowing him to bear the burdens of your stress is key to the management plan. Another key is to recognize red flags. Stressors recur and with practice you can recognize them and take action to defuse your response before it occurs.

Learn to Relax

A usual comment that I hear from patients is, "I just can't relax." Relaxing in a stressful situation is much easier for some than for others, but it is a learned behavior. We pattern many of our responses after the reactions we saw our parents or significant adults in our lives make when we were children. Even if those were destructive patterns, the dysfunction can stop with us. We don't have to respond in the same way.

Learn how to relax. Breathe deeply and slowly, let your tense muscles relax, take a break, and allow things to settle down. One technique for doing this is called progressive relaxation. Sit in a comfortable chair or on a couch.

Speak to each part of your body, beginning with your head and moving down to your toes, and allow it to relax. Playing soothing music while doing this is often helpful.

Getting your hair done, reading a book, getting a massage, or curling up in a comfortable chair and resting may be what you need to relax. Remember that it is okay to take some time for yourself. It will pay major dividends for you and your family, friends, and fellow workers.

Practice Acceptance

Learn to think through the stressful situation and carefully plan your response before you say or do anything. Most of us react in haste, and we often regret our responses.

It takes great maturity and self-control to step back from the issue at hand, weigh the possible responses, consider the effects on yourself and others, and then do what is right. God's Word tells us to treat others as we would have them treat us.

Remember that there are some things you cannot change. Friends, fellow workers, and your employer are all dealing with their own issues. Don't let their unwillingness to deal appropriately with events in their lives keep you from making decisions and choices that will bring wholeness to your life.

Evaluate Your Situation

I believe that job-related stress is one of the foremost issues confronting women. Some would prefer not to work but are forced into the work world because they are single or are single parents. They need the financial resources just to provide the basic essentials of life for themselves and for their families. Many women I speak with are resentful because they have to work when they would rather be at home with their children. If you don't absolutely have to work, and you are under stress because of your job, then seriously consider getting out of that situation.

You may also want to be certain that working is really a financially sound decision. In his book, *Money and Your Marriage*, Russ Crossen says, "I believe that the necessity for a mother to work in this way [contributing to the family's net income] will be seen as a myth if her actual contribution to the bottom line of the family's income is correctly calculated and analyzed."

Mothers, What's Your Paycheck Really Worth?

Salary	$10,000	$20,000	$30,000
Expenses			
Fixed			
Federal income tax[1]	1,500 (15%)	5,600 (28%)	8,400 (28%)
State income tax	600	1,200	1,800
Social Security tax	751	1,502	2,253
Tithe	1,000	2,000	3,000
Daycare credit[2]	(1,440)	(1,200)	(960)
Variable			
Transportation	600	600	600
Meals $2/day	480	480	480
Clothes	400	600	800
Hairdresser	300	400	500
Daycare (cash flow)[3]	6,240	6,240	6,240
Miscellaneous[4]	600	600	600
Total Expenses	(11,031)	(18,022)	(25,513)
Contribution to family income	($1,031)	$1,978	$6,487

1. 15% bracket if line 37 (taxable income on tax return) is less than $29,750; over $29,750 the bracket is 28%.
2. Credit equal to 30% of $2,400/child at $10,000 salary level and scaled down to 20% of $2,400/child at $30,000. Limited to 2 children.
3. 2 children at $65/week.
4. Convenience foods, forfeited savings on thrift shopping, etc.

In the chart on page 203, Crossen has calculated examples of the contribution to the family income of women who make annual salaries of $10,000, $20,000, and $30,000. Certain assumptions are listed in the footnotes to the chart.[1]

Analyze your financial situation and determine for yourself and your family whether the time and energy spent in a second job away from home is really worth it.

Get Organized

Being organized is another way to avoid stress. Some would say that developing lists and formulating plans for the day or week is stressful in itself, but in the long run, it is a good way to dissipate stress. When you have a plan of action, it prevents surges of anxiety that occur when you realize you have forgotten to do something or have not allowed enough time for an event.

Talk to Friends

Learn to communicate with others. Frequently a patient will describe to me in great detail some extremely stressful situation in her life. When I ask if she has talked to her husband or a friend about it, she will say, "No, he [or she] wouldn't understand anyway." Now I will grant you, there are many poor listeners among the male sex, but we can learn to be better communicators and listeners if you don't give up on us. Help us to learn how to help you. Recognize that we don't think the way you do; there is a physiologic block between our left and right brain hemispheres because of testosterone. Unless we are among those whose mothers helped them learn how to access the right side (feeling, empathy, and so forth), it is difficult for us. That is not an excuse; it is fact. Be a facilitator in this area, and it will benefit you in the long run.

Exercise

An essential part of stress management is physical exercise. First Corinthians 6:19 says that your body is a temple of God's Spirit. As such, you must care for it by keeping it clean and structurally sound. The foundation is obviously your personal relationship with Jesus. But staying sound physically is also a way in which we honor God's creation and it is crucial to dissipating stress.

The physical fitness craze has swept the United States, yet there are millions of Americans who ignore the condition of their body and wonder why they continue to feel unfit. A recent article in *Prevention* magazine, titled "The Prevention Index," indicated that only 30 percent of American women report that they do vigorous exercise frequently.[2]

Research has shown that a well-designed, appropriate exercise routine can favorably affect your emotional and physical responses to stress. The stress-induced outpouring of epinephrine and norepinephrine results in more rapid pulse, greater contractility of the heart, and higher blood pressure. Exercise, when done appropriately, results in release of *endorphins* (natural pain relievers) into the blood stream, producing a natural sense of well-being.

Endorphins also appear to burn up excess stress chemicals. Thus exercise enables you not only to metabolize the increased chemicals that are released by exercise, but also makes you more efficient in metabolizing those released by stress.

You may not think of yourself as an athlete. You don't have to be; just be willing to start exercising and persist diligently. It is important to slowly initiate a workout routine and build up your endurance. Don't wait until you have fibromyalgia or severe PMS to start; begin today. The benefits are well worth the effort and sweat.

Before you initiate your exercise program, you should have a complete physical examination. Your ultimate goal should be to exercise three to five times per week and to achieve 60 to 80 percent of your maximum predicted heart rate at the end of each twenty- to thirty-minute session (to find rate, subtract your age from 220; for example, if you are age 40, subtract 40 from 220, which leaves 180; 60 percent of 180 is 108, and 80 percent of 180 is 144; thus your target heart rate is 108–144 beats per minute). It will normally take six to twelve weeks to develop the endurance you need to achieve such a rate. Always stretch and warm up for five minutes before exercising. Before stopping, cool down for five minutes with a slowed rate of exercise.

Take it slow so you don't get discouraged. Initiating your program is the most difficult part. When you realize the benefits, you won't want to stop.

A form of exercise that emphasizes stress resolution and fitness was reported in the May 1994 issue of *American Health*. This form of mind-body fitness, developed by Carlos and Debbie Rosas in 1983, is called "neuro-muscular integrative action" (NIA). It is structured to be a slower, less intense workout than most conventional routines. The idea is to do stretches and calisthenics in a way that allows for individual creativity and expressivity in the choice of movements. By encouraging spontaneity, the mind remains focused on the workout and does not wander to thoughts of the stresses of the day.[3]

Eat Right

Diet is another essential aspect of stress management. You should eat sensibly. Well-balanced, calorie-appropriate meals are your best choice. Avoid fads and trends.

Just mention of the term *diet* to some people can result in an emotional outburst. Most women are not tall and slim, and they tire of being told that they must measure up to the standards set by models. After all, what type of routine or punishment does it take to maintain the lithe, hard-body look, and is it really beneficial to overall well-being? Remember, God looks at heart level, not physical appearance. He does intend for us to keep our temples fit, though. Good dietary habits alone will not make one healthy, but they certainly can play a major role in improving health if one suffers from any of the stress-associated disorders discussed in this book.

From my patients I believe that I have heard about every type of diet that has been tried. Should one restrict total calories or fat grams or carbohydrates or be a vegetarian or what? You can find a book or paper somewhere that would defend each of these principles. The best course is to eat a well-balanced, low-fat diet that is adequate in vitamins, minerals, amino acids, essential fatty acids, and energy sources. The neurotransmitter serotonin plays a critical role in an individual's mood. Increasing serotonin by dietary means or by using depressants, can improve mood and depressive symptoms. The best sources of serotonin are bananas and meat, especially turkey. Carbohydrates are necessary to enhance the absorption of serotonin by the body.

Some programs recommend herbal products. There are no good, well-designed, controlled studies to evaluate these preparations, but some holistic-medicine physicians feel that they are beneficial.

No, I am not going to prescribe a diet for you. I'm no fool! I want you to go on liking me. I would suggest that you see your own physician for a thorough physical examination and then consult a dietitian at your local clinic or hospital to get advice on the diet that is best suited to you.

There are many tables that indicate an appropriate weight according to height and age. Many of these have not been recently updated and may merely serve to depress. It is important to set realistic goals for weight loss or, if you are too thin, weight gain. It is also essential that behavior modification be incorporated into the program. A piece of paper with appropriate food selections written on it does not mean a thing unless you retrain your mind to believe the reasons for eating differently. You must understand the overall physical and emotional benefits.

Your brain carefully regulates your body weight at a specific level for you, called your set point. Unless you maintain your dietary and exercise programs, you will regain the weight you lose and return to your set-point weight. Data now indicate that you can reset your set point with continued exercise and a controlled diet.

Also remember that you will lose weight most rapidly at the beginning of the program, due to fluid loss and change in percent body fat. Don't get discouraged when the pounds come off more slowly later on. Keep at it. You can lose weight, and you will feel better for it.

Watch Your Habits

Although being physically unfit and overweight can cause tremendous medical and emotional problems, there is nothing more deleterious to your overall well-being than the abuse of nicotine, alcohol, caffeine, prescription drugs, or illegal drugs. Use of these agents gives one a temporary feeling of being in control of the situation. They are used to help cope with stress, but we know that the feeling is brief and then more substance is required.

It is currently estimated that fifty million Americans smoke cigarettes, cigars, or pipes. Unfortunately, the percentage of women who smoke has increased in recent years, in spite of numerous warnings against the adverse effects of active and passive inhalation of smoke. Ninety-eight percent of smokers are addicted to nicotine. One-third of all smokers will die as a direct result of their habit. Lung cancer is the second leading cancer killer of women.

Smoking increases the risk of developing pulmonary disease and cardiovascular disease. In pregnancy, nicotine not only increases the risk of complications for the mother but can adversely affect the unborn baby as well. Although no program to help people stop smoking can guarantee success, the best results are obtained in programs that combine education, behavior modification, and a withdrawal tool such as nicotine patches.

The use and abuse of alcohol continues to be a major problem among American women and men. One-third of all families in the United States experience a problem with alcohol abuse.

Are there any benefits of alcohol intake? Studies have shown that the daily intake of two ounces of alcohol is associated with increased longevity, possibly because of increases in high density lipoprotein cholesterol (HDL), which is the good form of cholesterol and protects blood vessels from plaque accumulation.

Unfortunately, a person has no idea if she has an addictive personality and may be unable to limit her drinking to two ounces a day. Women who have stress-related disorders may find it difficult to control their intake of anything that gives them a temporary sense of control of their stress.

Every individual has to determine what she will do. My advice is to avoid alcohol. If you are a problem drinker, I would strongly advise you to become involved with the Alcoholics Anonymous twelve-step program for recovery and to become active in your church. Don't wait until it is too late.

I would also encourage you to avoid caffeine as much as possible. Minimizing caffeine intake can improve the symptoms of fibrocystic breast disease, irritable bowel disease, and PMS.

Have Quiet Time

The last point about stress management is, I believe, the most essential to well-being—having a designated quiet time, a time to be alone, to study God's Word, to read insightful literature, to meditate and pray. God knows your deepest needs. His Spirit is ready and willing to come alongside you and minister to your spiritual and physical needs. He gives people moral freedom. God will not force himself upon you. You must give him permission to enter your life and be your stress resolver.

Making it a part of your regular schedule to take time alone is essential. Too many of us don't give God time to minister to us. Allow time for him to speak to you. You will find solace in your anguish over your stress-related disorders.

God has not given us a spirit of timidity, but of power and love and discipline.

2 Timothy 1:7

A Spiritual Perspective

Wherever you are in your life journey, whatever stressful situations you may be facing, I want to encourage you to open yourself up to the presence of God. Open your Bible to the psalms and begin reading until you find the very words that express the depths of your pain or problem. The Word of God is a balm to our wounded spirits, and it is healing for our brokenness. You do not need to be a biblical scholar to experience these benefits. Exercise your will and your God-given freedom to choose the way you will respond to the challenges that life presents. Let the difficulties you are facing at this very moment draw you into conversation with Christ. Perhaps you are reluctant to approach God because you have not done so in some time. You fear that he is waiting to get you, to judge and condemn you because you have not been a better Christian. Friends, this is simply a lie from the Enemy, who is the author of fear and distrust. God is waiting for you with open arms and a heart full of unconditional love. If you listen to the Enemy, he will keep your mind in fear and turmoil and anxiety, all designed to block you from receiving the healing love of God that is waiting for you.

Make sure there is no man or woman, clan or tribe among you today whose heart turns away from the LORD our God to go and worship the gods of those [other] nations; make sure there is no root among you that produces such bitter poison. When such a person hears the words of this

oath, he invokes a blessing on himself and therefore
thinks, "I will be safe, even though I persist in going my
own way." This will bring disaster on the watered land as
well as the dry.

Deuteronomy 29:18–19 NIV

As far back as Old Testament days, the tendency of humanity has been to look to someone or something other
than the one true God for help in time of need. In antiq-
uity, the people were accustomed to the worship of pagan
gods and found it difficult to lay down these old, albeit
unproductive, customs and place their total trust in the
one true God. In a pinch, they would run to their fertility
gods or storm gods, and as the writer of Deuteronomy
tells us, they would convince themselves that there would
be no harmful consequences of their actions. Are we any
different in contemporary society?

I want to suggest to you that at least a part of the stress
we experience comes to us because we insist on going our
own way, never consulting the Lord for wisdom or direction. We are ignorant of what the Word tells us will be the
inevitable consequences: disaster.

Deuteronomy 29:19 says this kind of disobedience will
"bring disaster on the watered land and the dry." In other
words, the ripple effect of our rebellion has the very real
potential to bring difficulties into our lives, in areas where
we think we have our act together (the watered land) as
well as into those areas where we are struggling (dry land).
This kind of disobedience puts our backs to the Lord and
our eyes on our problems. It has been my experience that
at this point God will wait for us to make a move. But our
loving heavenly Father is seeking to get our attention in
every possible way. Consequently he will allow the logi-
cal consequences of our choices to have their reign in our

lives. Many times we have to experience deep suffering before we are desperate enough to go God's way. God loves us enough to allow this "severe mercy" into our lives. In time, if we will allow it, this severe mercy will do a work of grace in us that mere kindness could never do. As we finally turn back to him in the midst of our deepest pain, we find his unconditional love waiting to embrace us.

Now look at Isaiah 26:3. When we choose to focus our thought life on God and his resources instead of focusing primarily on our problems, the consequence is peace—perfect peace. Isaiah goes on to describe God as the "Rock eternal" (v. 4 NIV). This kind of perfect peace is the exact opposite of stress. It is available to us from only one resource: God the Father, through his Son Jesus, by the supernatural power of the Holy Spirit.

The book of 2 Timothy offers us encouragement. Paul is writing some of his last words from prison as he nears certain death. Even though he is "chained like a criminal," Paul declares, "God's word is not chained" (2:9 NIV). Paul was suffering, facing death, but he did not wallow in self-pity. Read the entire book of 2 Timothy (it's a very short book) to see where Paul turned for help.

Let's focus our attention for a moment on those wonderful words of the first chapter, at verses 6 and 7. Paul's words form the basis of my challenge to you: "Fan into flame the gift of God, which is in you. . . . for God did not give us a spirit of timidity [fear], but a spirit of power, of love and of self-discipline" (NIV). While our hearts are bent down in humility at the knowledge of our own unworthiness, because of what Jesus did for us on the cross, we can nonetheless move with boldness and assurance into the presence of the one true God. Jesus' death and temporary separation from God tore down the walls that used to separate us from the Father and made it possible for anyone who calls on Jesus as Savior to gain access to all the heavenly resources we could ever need.

The Lord stands ready and more willing than we can ever know to meet us at the point of our deepest need. Will you trust him? Step off the banks and move into the ongoing river of his love.

Jesus will transform your turmoil into your tool and equip you with every resource you will need to meet the challenges that are an inevitable part of life.

My recipe for stress relief: One part repentance to immeasurable parts of grace and mercy. Many cups of bitter sorrow to one drop of redeeming blood from the brow of our Savior. Combine all of these ingredients with the breath of life and the integrity of the human capacity for choice. Mix with generous doses of prayer and bake in the purifying fire of the love of God for as long as it takes to get it done. Prepare fresh daily and serve warm.

Notes

Chapter 1 What Is Stress and How Does It Affect You?

1. Hans Seyle, *The Stress of Life* (New York: McGraw Hill, 1956), 1–14.

2. Juliet Schor, *The Overworked American* (New York: Basic Books, 1992), 1–15.

3. Hans Selye, *Stress in Health and Disease* (Boston: Butterworth, 1976), 725–895.

4. Neil S. Hibler, "Making the Best of Stress," *Airman* (1981).

5. Robert S. Eliot and Dennis L. Breo, *Is It Worth Dying For?* (New York: Bantam, 1989), 36–55.

6. Ibid, 28–31.

Chapter 2 The Stress of Abuse

1. Dean G. Kilpatrick et al., "The Aftermath of Rape: Recent Empirical Findings," *American Journal of Orthopsychiatry* 49 (1979): 658–69.

2. D. G. Kilpatrick, L. Veronen, and P. Resnick, "Assessment of the Aftermath of Rape: Changing Patterns of Fear," *Journal of Behavioral Assessment* (1980): 327–31.

3. Judith Herman, *Trauma and Recovery* (New York: Basic Books, 1992), 157–58, 211–13.

4. Ellen Bass and Laura Davis, *The Courage to Heal: A Guide for Women Survivors of Child Sexual Abuse* (New York: HarperCollins, 1988), 118–21.

Chapter 3 Premenstrual Syndrome

1. R. L. Reid and S. S. C. Yen, "Premenstrual Syndrome," *American Journal of Obstetrics and Gynecology* 139 (1981): 85–104.

2. American Psychiatric Association, *Diagnostic and Statistical Manual of Mental Disorders,* 4th ed. (Washington, D.C.: American Psychiatric Press, 1994), 715–16.

3. L. E. Beck, R. Gevirtz, and J. F. Mortola, "The Predictive Role of Psychosocial Stress on Symptom Severity in Premenstrual Syndrome," *Psychosomatic Medicine* 52 (1990): 536–43; and L. Gannon et al., "Perimenstrual Symptoms: Relationships with Chronic Stress and Selected Lifestyle Variables," *Behavioral Medicine* 15 (1989): 149–59.

4. A. B. Heilbrun Jr. and M. E. Frank, "Self-preoccupation and General Stress Level as Sensitizing Factors in Premenstrual and Menstrual Distress," *Journal of Psychosomatic Research* 33, no. 5 (1989): 571–77.

5. Carol Tavris, *The Mismeasure of Women* (New York: Simon and Schuster, 1992), 131–55.

6. D. Avery, "Dawn Simulation Treatment of Winter Depression: A Controlled Study," *American Journal of Psychiatry* 150 (1993): 113–17.

Chapter 5 Headaches

1. O. Hallesby, *Prayer* (Minneapolis: Augsburg, 1994), 14.
2. Ibid, 15.

Chapter 6 Irritable Bowel Syndrome

1. "Communion Ritual," *The Methodist Hymnal* (Nashville: Whitmore and Smith, 1939), 506.

Chapter 7 Fibromyalgia

1. D. L. Goldenberg, D. T. Felson, and H. Dinerman, "A Randomized Controlled Trial of Amitriptyline and Naproxen in the Treatment of Patients with Fibromyalgia," *Arthritis Rheumatology* 29 (1986): 1371–77.

2. H. A. Smythe and H. Moldofsky, "Two Contributions to the Understanding of the 'Fibrositis' Syndrome," *Bulletin of Rheumatic Disease* 28 (1977): 928–31.

3. Paul Davidson, *Chronic Muscle Pain Syndrome* (Philadelphia: Villard Books, 1990).

Chapter 10 Eating Disorders

1. J. E. Brown, "Influence of Pregnancy Weight Gain," *Obstetrics and Gynecology* 57 (1981): 13–17.

2. S. Sohlberg, "Personality, Life Stress and the Course of Eating Disorders," *Acta Psychiatrica* 361 (1990): 29–33.

3. R. G. Laessie et al., "A Comparison of Nutritional Management with Stress Management in the Treatment of Bulimia Nervosa," *British Journal of Psychiatry* 159 (1991): 250–61.

4. Laura Humphreys, "You Think a Friend Has a Eating Disorder: What Should You Do?" (University of Kentucky Medical School Eating Disorders Clinic, patient handout).

Chapter 11 Substance Abuse

1. A. B. McBride, "Multiple Roles," *Women's Mental Health Research Agenda* (Rockville, Md.: National Institute of Mental Health, 1988), 33–37.

2. L. A. Pohorecky, "Stress and Alcohol Interaction: An Update of Human Research," *Alcohol and Clinical Experience for the Resident* 15 (1991): 438–59.

Chapter 12 Skin Disorders

1. J. Y. Koo and C. T. Pham, "Psychodermatology: Practical Guidelines on Pharmacotherapy," *Archives of Dermatology* 128 (1992): 381–88.

Chapter 14 Stress Resolution Guidelines

1. Russ Crossen, *Money and Your Marriage* (Atlanta: Ronald Blue and Co., 1989), 76.

2. "The Prevention Index 1995," *Prevention* , 3.

3. D. Eller, "Workouts That Fight Stress," *American Health* 5 (1994): 72–77.

Bibliography

American Psychiatric Association. *Diagnostic and Statistical Manual of Mental Disorders.* 4th ed. Washington, D.C.: American Psychiatric Press, 1994.

Avery, D. "Dawn Simulation Treatment of Winter Depression: A Controlled Study." *American Journal of Psychiatry* 150 (1993): 113–17.

Baltrusch, H. J., W. Stangel, and I. Titze. "Stress, Cancer and Immunity: New Developments in Biopsychosocial and Psychoneuroimmunologic Research." *Acta Neurologica* 13 (1991): 315–27.

Bass, Ellen, and Laura Davis. *The Courage to Heal: A Guide for Women Survivors of Child Sexual Abuse.* New York: HarperCollins, 1988.

Beaton, R. D., et al. "Self-Reported Symptoms of Stress with Temporomandibular Disorders: Comparisons to Healthy Men and Women." *Journal of Prosthetic Dentistry* 65, no. 2 (1991): 289–93.

Beck, L. E., R. Gevirtz, and S. F. Mortola, "The Predictive Role of Psychosocial Stress on Symptom Severity in Premenstrual Syndrome." *Psychosomatic Medicine* 52 (1990): 536–43.

Bennett, R. M. "Fibrositis: Does It Exist and Can It Be Treated?" *Journal of Musculoskeletal Medicine* 1, no. 7 (1984): 57–72.

Benson, H. *The Relaxation Response.* New York: William Morrow and Co., 1975.

Biety, J. R., J. H. Williford Jr., and E. A. McMullen. "Alcohol Craving in Rehabilitation: Assessment of Nutrition Therapy." *Journal of the American Dietary Association* 91 (1991): 463–66.

Blanchard, E. B., et al. "The Role of Anxiety and Depression in the Irritable Bowel Syndrome." *Behavioral Research and Therapy* 28 (1990): 401–5.

Blau, J. N. "Migraine Triggers: Practice and Therapy." *Pathology and Biology* 40 (1992): 367–72.

Born, W., R. Harbeck, and R. L. O'Brien. "Possible Links between the Immune System and Stress Response: The Role of Gamma Delta T-Lymphocytes." *Semin Immunol* 3 (1991): 443–48.

Brown, J. E. "Influence of Pregnancy Weight Gain." *Obstetrics and Gynecology* 57 (1981): 13–17.

Chaterton, R. T. "The Role of Stress in Female Reproduction: Animal and Human Considerations." *International Journal of Fertility* 35 (1990): 8–13.

Claus, K. E., and J. T. Bailey. *Living with Stress and Promoting Well-Being.* St. Louis: C. V. Mosby, 1980.

Crossen, Russ. *Money and Your Marriage.* Atlanta: Ronald Blue and Co., 1989.

Dalton, K. *The Premenstrual Syndrome and Progesterone Therapy.* 2d ed. Chicago: Year Book Medical, 1984.

Davidson, P. *Chronic Muscle Pain Syndrome.* Philadelphia: Villard Books, 1990.

DeBenedittis, G., and A. Lorenzetti. "The Role of Stressful Life Events in the Persistence of Primary Headache: Major Events vs. Daily Hassles. *Pain* 51 (1992): 35–42.

DeBenedittis, G., A. Lorenzetti, and A. Pieri. "The Role of Stressful Life Events in the Onset of Chronic Primary Headache." *Pain* 40 (1990): 65–75.

"Depression in Women," *ACOG Technical Bulletin* 182 (July 1993).

Dinning, W. D., and A. M. Guptil. "Jenkins Type A Scores in the Relation of Stress and Premenstrual Symptoms." *Psychol Rep* 70 (1992): 1152–54.

Duffle, N. *Helpful Habits for Intestinal Health.* Cincinnati: On Target Media, Inc.

Eliot, Robert S., and Dennis L. Breo. *Is It Worth Dying For?* New York: Bantam, 1989.

Eller, D. "Workouts That Fight Stress." *American Health* 5 (1994): 72–77.

Ellis, L. F., L. D. Black, and P. A. Resick. "The Cognitive-Behavioral Treatment Approaches for Victims of Crime." *Innovations in Clinical Practice: A Source Book,* vol. 11, 1992.

Engel, B. *The Right to Innocence: Healing the Trauma of Childhood Sexual Abuse.* New York: Ivy Books, 1989.

Fan, P. T., and M. E. Blanton. "Clinical Features and Diagnosis of Fibromyalgia." *Journal of Musculoskeletal Medicine* 9 (1992): 24–42.

Frank, R. T. "The Hormonal Basis of Premenstrual Tension." *Archives of Neurology and Psychiatry* 26 (1931): 1053–57.

Gannon, et al. "Perimenstrual Symptoms: Relationships with Chronic Stress and Selected Life Style Variables." *Behavioral Medicine* 15 (1989): 149–59.

Gil, Eliana. *Outgrowing the Pain: A Book for and about Adults Abused as Children.* San Francisco: Launch Press, 1983.

Gilbert, S. "Your Period: What's Normal, What's Not." *Redbook,* September 1992, 32–36.

Gilliotte, B. W. *Fibromyalgia: A Patient Primer.* The Fibromyalgia Group.

Girdans, D., and E. George. *Controlling Stress and Tension: A Holistic Approach.* Englewood Cliffs, N.J.: Prentice-Hall, 1979.

Goldenberg, D. L., D. T. Felson, and H. Dinerman. "A Randomized Controlled Trial of Amitriptyline and Naproxen in the Treatment of Patients with Fibromyalgia." *Arthritis Rheumatology* 29 (1986): 1371-77.

Greene, R., and K. Dalton. "The Premenstrual Syndrome." *British Medical Journal* 1 (1953): 1007–14.

Guthrie, E., et al. "A Controlled Trial of Psychological Treatment for the Irritable Bowel Syndrome." *Gastroenterology* 100 (1991): 450–57.

Hallesby, O. *Prayer.* Minneapolis: Augsburg, 1994.

Harlow, S. D., and G. M. Matanoski. "The Association between Weight, Physical Activity and Stress and Variation in the Length of the Menstrual Cycle." *American Journal of Epidemiology* 133 (1991): 39–49.

Heilbrun, A. B., Jr., and M. E. Frank. "Self-preoccupation and General Stress Level as Sensitizing Factors in Premenstrual and Menstrual Distress." *Journal of Psychosomatic Research* 33, no. 5 (1989): 571–77.

Herman, Judith L. *Trauma and Recovery.* New York: Basic Books, 1992.

Hibler, Neil S. "Making the Best of Stress." *Airman,* 1981.

Holroyd, K. A., et al. "A Comparison of Pharmacological (Amitriptyline HCI) and Nonpharmacological (Cognitive-Behavioral) Therapies for Chronic Tension Headaches." *Journal of Consulting Clinical Psychologists* 59 (1991): 387–93.

Jankovic, B. D. "Neuro-Immune Network: Basic Structural and Functional Correlates." *Acta Neurologica* 13 (1991): 305–14.

Josephs, R. A., and C. M. Steele. "The Two Faces of Alcohol Myopia: Attentional Mediation of Psychological Stress." *Journal of Abnormal Psychology* 99 (1990): 115–26.

Kellow, J. E., et al. "Effects of Acute Psychologic Stress on Small Intestinal Motility in Health and the Irritable Bowel Syndrome." *Scandinavian Journal of Gastroenterology* 27 (1992): 53–58.

Kessler, R. C., et al. "Affective Disorders Lifetime Prevalence: Men vs. Women." *Archives of General Psychiatry* 51 (1994): 8–19.

Khansari, D. N., A. J. Murgo, and R. E. Faith. "Effects of Stress on the Immune System." *Immunology Today* 11 (1990): 170–75.

Kilpatrick, D. G., et al. "The Aftermath of Rape: Recent Empirical Findings." *American Journal of Orthopsychiatry* 49 (1979): 658–69.

Kilpatrick, D. G., L. Veronen, and P. Resnick. "Assessment of the Aftermath of Rape: Changing Patterns of Fear." *Journal of Behavioral Assessment* (1980): 327–31.

Kohler, T., and C. Haimerl. "Daily Stress as a Trigger of Migraine Attacks: Results of Thirteen Single-Subject Studies." *Consultant in Clinical Psychology* 58 (1990): 870–72.

Koo, J. Y., and C. T. Pham. "Psychodermatology: Practical Guidelines on Pharmacotherapy." *Archives of Dermatology* 128 (1992): 381–88.

Laessie, R. G., et al. "A Comparison of Nutritional Management with Stress Management in the Treatment of Bulimia Nervosa." *British Journal of Psychiatry* 159 (1991): 250–61.

Lance, J. W. "Headache." *Annals of Neurology* 10 (1981): 1–10.

Lefebvre, R. C., and S. L. Sandford. "A Multi-Model Questionnaire for Stress." *Journal of Human Stress* 11 (1985): 69–75.

Lex, B. "Gender Differences and Substance Abuse." In *Advances in Substance Abuse, Behavioral and Biological Research*. Ed. N. K. Mello. London: Jessica Kingsley Press, 1991.

McBride, A. B. "Multiple Roles." *Women's Mental Health Research Agenda.* Women's Mental Health Occasional Paper Series. Rockville, Md.: National Institute of Mental Health, 1988, 33–37.

Mannheimer, J. S., and R. M. Rosenthal. "Acute and Chronic Postural Abnormalities as Related to Craniofacial Pain and Temporomandibular Disorders." *Dental Clinics of North America* 35, no. 1 (1991): 185–208.

Marshall, M. "Stress Management in Dermatology Patients." *Nursing Standard* 5 (1991): 29–31.

Mithers, C. L. "Stress Sex." *Ladies Home Journal,* September 1993, 62–72.

Moschella, S. L. *Dermatology.* 3d ed. Philadelphia: W. B. Saunders Co., 1992.

Musek, "Hormonal Manipulation in the Treatment of Premenstrual Syndrome," *Clinics in Obstetrics and Gynecology* 35 (1991): 658–66.

Myburgh, K. H., et al. "Low Bone Density Is an Etiologic Factor for Stress Fractures in Athletes." *Annals of Internal Medicine* 113 (1990): 754–59.

National Institute of Mental Health. "Eating Disorders." Washington, D.C.: NIH Publication, no. 93 (1993): 3477.

O'Doherty, F. "Is Drug Use a Response to Stress?" *Drug and Alcohol Dependency* 29 (1991): 97–106.

O'Leary, A. "Stress, Emotion and Human Immune Function." *Psychology Bulletin* 108 (1990): 363–82.

Ottaway, C. A., and A. J. Husband. "Central Nervous System Influences on Lymphocyte Migration." *Brain Behavior and Immunology* 6 (1992): 97–116.

Passchier, J., P. Goudswaard, and Orlebeke. "Abnormal Extracranial Vasomotor Response in Migraine Sufferers to Real-Life Stress." *Psychosomatic Research* 37 (1993): 405–14.

Pear, M. J. "When the Aches and Pains Aren't Arthritis." *Nations Business,* 1990, 70.

Pingitore, G., V. Chrobak, and J. Petrie. "The Social and Psychologic Factors of Bruxism." *Journal of Prosthetic Dentistry* 65, no. 3 (1991): 443–46.

Plouffe, L., Jr., et al. "Premenstrual Syndrome: Update on Diagnosis and Management." *The Female Patient* 19 (1994): 53–60.

Pohorecky, L. A. "Stress and Alcohol Interaction: An Update of Human Research." *Alcohol and Clinical Experience for the Resident* 15 (1991): 438–59.

Quinn, J. H. "Arthroscopic and Histologic Evidence of Chondromalacia in the Temporomandibular Joint." *Oral Surgery Oral Medicine Oral Pathology* 70, no. 3 (1990): 387–92.

Rasmussen, B. K. "Migraine and Tension-Type Headache in a General Population: Precipitating Factors, Female Hormones, Sleep Pattern and Relation to Lifestyle." *Pain* 53 (1993): 65–72.

Reid, R. L., and S. S. C. Yen. "Premenstrual Syndrome." *American Journal of Obstetrics and Gynecology* 139 (1981): 85–104.

Rhodes, J. E., and L. A. Jason. "A Social Stress Model of Substance Abuse." *Journal of Consulting Clinical Psychologists* 58 (1990): 395–401.

Root, M. P., et al. *Bulimia: A Systems Approach to Treatment.* New York: W. W. Norton and Co., 1986.

Rosenthal, N. E. "The Treatment of Seasonal Affective Disorders." *Journal of the American Medical Association* 270 (1993): 2717–20.

Schenker, J., D. Meirow, and E. Schenker. "Stress and Human Reproduction." *European Journal of Obstetrics Gynecology and Reproductive Biology* 45 (1992): 1–8.

Schor, Juliet B. *The Overworked American.* New York: Basic Books, 1992.

Schroeder, H., et al. "Causes and Signs of Temporomandibular Joint Pain and Dysfunction: An Electromyographical Investigation." *Oral Rehabilitation* 18, no. 4 (1991): 301–10.

Schwarz, S. P., et al. "Psychological Aspects of Irritable Bowel Syndrome: Comparisons with Inflammatory Bowel Disease and Nonpatient Controls." *Behavioral Research Therapy* 31 (1993): 297–304.

Seyle, Hans. *The Stress of Life.* New York: McGraw Hill, 1956.

———. *Stress in Health and Disease.* Boston: Butterworth, 1976.

Shaw, G., et al. "Stress Management for Irritable Bowel Syndrome: A Controlled Trial." *Digestion* 50 (1991): 36–42.

Sherman, C. "Stressed Out or Really Sick? How to Tell." *McCall's*, November 1992.

Smith, E. M., C. R. Cloninger, and S. Bradford. "Predictors of Mortality in Alcoholic Women: A Prospective Followup Study." *Alcoholism: Clinical Experimental Research* 7 (1983): 237–43.

Smythe, H. A., and H. Moldofsky. "Two Contributions to the Understanding of the 'Fibrositis' Syndrome." *Bulletin of Rheumatic Disease* 28 (1977): 928–31.

Sohlberg, S. "Personality, Life Stress and the Course of Eating Disorders." *Acta Psychiatrica* 361 (1990): 29–33.

Soukup, V. M., M. E. Beiler, and F. Terrell. "Stress, Coping Style, and Problem Solving Ability among Eating-Disordered Inpatients." *Journal of Clinical Psychology* 46 (1990): 592–99.

Stress Management: Ten Self-Care Techniques in Innovations in Clinical Practice: A Source Book. Vol. 5, 427–29.

Taddey J. J. "Rationale for Sequential Use of Both Maxillary and Mandibular Orthopedic Appliances in the Treatment of TMJ Disorders." *Journal of Craniomandibular Disorders* 4, no. 4 (1990): 273–75.

Tavris, Carol. *The Mismeasure of Women.* New York: Simon and Schuster, 1992.

Ussher, J. M., and J. M. Wilding. "Performance and State Changes During the Menstrual Cycle, Conceptualized within a Broad Band Testing Framework." *Social Science and Medicine* 32 (1991): 525–34.

Uveges, J. M., et al. "Psychological Symptoms in Primary Fibromyalgia Syndrome: Relationship to Pain, Life Stress and Sleep Disturbances." *Arthritis Theum* 33 (1990): 1279–83.

VanThiel, D. H., and J. S. Gavaler. "Ethanol Metabolism and Hepatotoxicity: Does Sex Make a Difference?" In *Recent Developments in Alcoholism.* Edited by M. Galanter. New York: Plenum Press, 1988, 291–304.

Walters, V. "Women's Views of Their Main Health Problems." *Canadian Journal of Public Health* 83 (1992): 371–74.

Weinberger, M., et al. "Social Support, Stress and Functional Status in Patient with Osteoarthritis." *Social Science Medicine* 30 (1990): 503–8.

Whitehead, W. E., et al. "Effects of Stressful Life Events on Bowel Symptoms: Subjects with Irritable Bowel Syndrome Compared with Subjects without Bowel Dysfunction." *Gut* 33 (1992): 825–30.

Whorwell, P. J., et al. "Physiological Effects of Emotion: Assessment via Hypnosis." *Lancet* 340 (1992): 69–72.

Yanovski, S. Z. "Binge Eating Disorder: Current Knowledge and Future Directions." *Obesity Research* 1 (1993): 306–24.